Pulmonary Function Testing
&
Interpretation

Pulmonary Function Testing & Interpretation

James E Hansen MD FACP FCCP APS ATS

Emeritus Professor of Medicine
David Geffen UCLA School of Medicine
Respiratory and Critical Care Physiology and Medicine
Los Angeles Biomedical Research Institute
at Harbor-UCLA Medical Center
Torrance, CA, USA

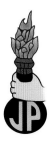

JAYPEE BROTHERS MEDICAL PUBLISHERS (P) LTD

New Delhi • Panama City • London

Jaypee Brothers Medical Publishers (P) Ltd.

Headquarters

Jaypee Brothers Medical Publishers (P) Ltd
4838/24, Ansari Road, Daryaganj
New Delhi 110 002, India
Phone: +91-11-43574357
Fax: +91-11-43574314
Email: jaypee@jaypeebrothers.com

J.P. Medical Ltd.,
83 Victoria Street London
SW1H 0HW (UK)
Phone: +44-2031708910
Fax: +02-03-0086180
Email: info@jpmedpub.com

Jaypee-Highlights Medical Publishers Inc.
City of Knowledge, Bld. 237, Clayton
Panama City, Panama
Phone: 507-317-0160
Fax: +50-73-010499
Email: cservice@jphmedical.com

Website: www.jaypeebrothers.com
Website: www.jaypeedigital.com

© 2011, Jaypee Brothers Medical Publishers

Inquiries for bulk sales may be solicited at: jaypee@jaypeebrothers.com

This book has been published in good faith that the contents provided by the author(s) contained herein are original, and is intended for educational purposes only. While every effort is made to ensure a accuracy of information, the publisher and the author(s) specifically disclaim any damage, liability, or loss incurred, directly or indirectly, from the use or application of any of the contents of this work. If not specifically stated, all figures and tables are courtesy of the authors(s). Where appropriate, the readers should consult with a specialist or contact the manufacturer of the drug or device.

Publisher: Jitendar P Vij
Publishing Director: Tarun Duneja
Editors: Naren Aggarwal, Shaila Prashar
Cover Design: Seema Dogra, Sachin Dhawan

Clinical Focus Series
Pulmonary Function Testing & Interpretation
First Edition: **2011**

ISBN-13: 978-93-5025-105-8

Printed at Replika Press Pvt. Ltd.

PREFACE

It was an honor to be asked by Jaypee Brothers and is a pleasure to write this monograph on pulmonary physiology laboratory testing and interpretation. The lungs and heart share the thorax for good reasons. We are reminded that our knowledge and understanding of the structure and the function of the human respiratory and circulatory systems is recent. Pulmonary laboratory findings can help us better identify and quantify dysfunction in individuals damaged by multiple factors or exposure to hazardous particulates, allergens, and chemicals, including cigarette smoke. Laboratory findings can help physicians in the diagnosis and care of these patients.

Although some of the data presented and my opinions may be controversial or even heretical, I hope you will consider the accompanying analyses, discussions, and recommendations. Please note especially the presentation of new reference equations for spirometry, lung volumes, and gas transfer, applicable for the entire earth's adult population, i.e., the minority "whites (W)" and the majority "others (M)".

May I express my appreciation to the following individuals who have influenced me positively:

1. Stimulating high school teachers, especially Genevieve Bender, Donald McMaster, and Lawrence McPhail;
2. College and medical school colleagues, especially Jeremiah Barondess, Pierce Flynn, William Fritz, Donald Fry, Benjamin Gaston, William Insull, Dwight McGoon, Victor McKusick, Gilbert Mellin, Howard Morgan, Ronald Seaton, and Arthur Siemens;
3. Faculty at Johns Hopkins, especially A McGehee Harvey, Joseph Lilienthal, Arnold Rich, and Helen Taussig;
4. Many fine physicians during my military service, especially Ted Bacharach, J Edward Canham, Harry Dean, Robert Dickerson, L Howard Hartley, Leroy Jones, Robert C Jones, Eddy D Palmer, Marjorie and Bill Sirridge, and George Woodard;
5. Role models, mentors, and colleagues in Denver, especially Frank Consolazio, Giles Filley, Robert Grover, J Patrick Hannon, and Wiltz Wagner;
6. Role models, mentors, and colleagues at UCLA, especially Yo Aelony, Richard Casaburi, Dick Effros, Gregory Hirsch, David Hsia, Greg Mason, Paul Selecky,

Kathy Sietsema, Darryl Sue, Xing-Guo Sun, William Stringer, Donald Tashkin, Donald Tierney, Janine Vintch, Herbert Webb, Brain Whipp, and above all, Karlmann Wasserman;

7. Interns, residents, and fellows at Harbor-UCLA Medical Center, dedicated and talented physicians, too numerous to individually identify;

8. Laboratory personnel at Harbor-UCLA Medical Center, especially Doctors Solita Ong, Terry Robinson, and Aiping Zhou; and David Adame, Chul Ki Hong, Raymund Adoc, and Cesar Siguenza,

9. Pulmonary physiologists elsewhere, especially Jack Clausen, Robert Crapo, and Antonius Van Kessel;

10. Nico and Ellen Smith, a South African theologian and psychiatrist who courageously overthrew apartheid;

11. Friends who battled against homelessness, especially Emmitt Blankenfeld, Clayton Cobb, John Copper, Steve English, Darryl Floyd, Ruth Lohrer, and Bob Pratt; and

12. Brave members of our Armed Forces who sacrificed so much during WWII, the Korean War, and the Vietnam War, while I was on active duty as a student and physician. I had the opportunity to work with dedicated US Army personnel in the treatment of tens of thousands of these courageous men and women as patients, although I escaped the dangers and hardships they endured.

Importantly, my love and gratitude to:

- Helen Terp and Jim Hansen, my inspiring parents;
- John, Muriel, David, and Paul, my talented siblings;
- Evelyn and Harvey Kapke, generous parents of my wife;
- Beverly Kapke Hansen; my supportive (and beautiful) wife and best friend;
- Our accomplished children and their spouses, Barbara and Karl, Patricia and Kevin, Linda and Chris, and Ann and Jim, and their fine children.

Finally, I appreciate the encouragement and expertise of Dr Naren Aggarwal and his staff at Jaypee Brothers. The mistakes and errors in this publication are mine. I welcome your comments, whether supportive or not.

James E Hansen

CONTENTS

1 History of Respiratory Physiology

INTRODUCTION

Where references are not specifically documented, the details in this chapter are extracted from John F. Perkins Jr's. excellent presentation.[1] It is not necessary for you to read this brief *history* of respiration and the role of the pulmonary and cardiovascular systems. However, *this story* makes us grateful for the brilliance and insights of our forebearers who made great progress despite the limited technology available to them. History also reminds us of the difficulties in changing others' opinions and concepts when new facts conflict with widely held beliefs. We must ask: "Which of our current beliefs and practices will be found to be false in the near and distant future?"

ANCIENT KNOWLEDGE

It is clear that the ancient Egyptians of 3000 BCE, Chinese of 2000 BCE and Hebrews of 1000 BCE had some knowledge of bodily functions, diseases, and medical and surgical treatments, but little is known of their understanding of respiration. Genesis, chapter 2, verse 7, states, "Then the Lord God formed man (Adam) from the dust of the ground, and breathed into his nostrils the breath of life; and man became a living being."[2] At about 550 BCE, Anaximenes of Asia Minor stated, "As our soul, being air, sustains us, so pneumo (breath) and air pervade the whole world". Empedocles of Sicily at about 450 BCE theorized that blood ebbing and flowing from the heart distributed "innate heat" to the body, that respiration took place through the skin and the lungs, and that the four essential elements of matter were earth, air, fire and water. Diogenes of the same era believed that blood vessels carried air throughout the body.

Hippocrates and his colleagues in approximately 400 BCE described tuberculosis, friction rubs and signs of pleural effusions. Hippocrates, Plato, and Aristotle (384-348 BCE) all believed that the heart was the seat of innate heat and that the purpose of respiration was to cool the heart. The atria acted as bellows to push air from the pulmonary vein to the left ventricle and from the pulmonary artery to the right ventricle. Although Aristotle had dissected many animals, he located the seat of intelligence in the heart, a belief which persisted for many centuries. His philosophical beliefs conflicted with those of Democritus (400 BCE) who believed in mechanistic and deterministic causes of living things.

About 300 BCE, veins were distinguished from arteries; the latter were believed to contain air (Most bodies examined post-mortem were likely victims of violent deaths and relatively void of blood). Erasistratus (~250 BCE) proposed a pneumatic theory of respiration, with air distributed through arteries, veins and hollow nerves. Galen (130-199 CE) often called the "father of anatomy", performed several public human dissections. He apparently proposed three "pneumata" or life-giving "spirits" which were added to blood: "natural spirit" from the liver, "vital spirit" which could pass through invisible pores between the ventricles, and a later named "animal spirit" originating in the brain and transmitted through hollow nerves. Galen attacked Aristotle's belief that the heart was the seat of the sensitive soul. He showed that nerves originated in the brain; the chordae tendineae were not nerves; the phrenic nerve enervated the diaphragm; the function of the recurrent pharyngeal nerve; and that sound was caused by vibrations of air. After Galen's death, the study of anatomy and physiology ceased in Europe, so that only his views were taught there until the 17th century!

DARK AGES AND EARLY RENAISSANCE

Many Arabic scientists and physicians had different views challenging Galen's views, but the burning of the library at Alexandria in 391 CE by Christian fanatics destroyed many priceless works including their findings. In the 12th and 13th centuries some Arabic works were translated into Latin, influencing many European scholars including Roger Bacon (1192-1280), who was imprisoned for his advanced beliefs. For example, Ibn An-Nafis of Damascus (1210-1288) described the course of blood from the right side of the heart through the lungs to the left heart, not through Galen's pores in the ventricles.

Leonardo da Vinci (1452-1519) made superlative anatomical (and mechanical) drawings. He confirmed that the lungs were expanded by movements of the thorax and that it was impossible for air to reach the interior of the heart. Andreas Vesalius (1514-1564), perhaps the foremost anatomist of all time, noted the absence of pores between the ventricles and described the lung very well, including the courses of the pulmonary arteries and veins but not the movement of blood in the lungs. He also conducted extensive physiological studies on living animals but was denounced as a madman and driven out of academic work since his findings did not conform to those of Galen. Michael Servitus (1511-1553), a Spanish theologian and anatomist, published a thousand copies of his book which were nearly all destroyed by fanatics. He described the flow of blood from the right heart to the left heart, adding that the blood changed color in its journey through the lung. He did not describe the systemic flow of blood or use the "circle" word. His views were considered so heretical by both Catholics and Protestants that he was burned at the stake in Geneva!

William Harvey (1578-1657), called the father of physiology, fortunately lived much longer, and described well the flow of blood in one direction in the systemic and pulmonary circle. He believed that movements of the lung were indispensable for the circulation of blood through them, but questioned whether the lungs heated or cooled, or otherwise altered the blood.

FIFTEENTH THROUGH EIGHTEENTH CENTURIES

Microscopic anatomy and chemistry were unknown to Harvey and his immediate colleagues. In Bologna, Marcello Malpighi (1628-1694) washed and dried animal lungs, inflated them through the trachea, and with his microscope, described the flask-shaped structures of alveoli and lung capillaries and the separation of blood from air! Later he described the capillary circulation of the mesentery and concluded for the first time that blood was not forced into open spaces but was always within tubules, later named "capillaries". Giovanni Borelli (1608-1679), who must have understood much of respiration, drafted descriptions of equipment which might be used for underwater diving, with snorkels or goatskins to supply air, and a bronze helmet with glass window.

Four British scientists [Robert Boyle (1627-1691), Robert Hooke (1635-1703), Richard Lower (1631-1691), and John Mayow (1643-1679)] made major advances in respiratory physiology. They realized that: (a) fresh air was necessary for life; (b) air under increased pressure was better in this regard than ordinary air; (c) air in lungs changed the color of blood to bright red; (d) the new insight that "nitro-aerial" spirit (i.e., a portion of the air) was necessary for both combustion and respiration and (e) metals could decrease or increase in weight after burning or heating.

Further understanding of combustion and metabolism was sidetracked by GE Stahl (1660-1734) who theorized that the substance phlogiston, which could be burned, existed in all things. It was difficult to overcome his well-accepted theory. Joseph Black (1728-1790) discovered "fixed air" (e.g., later found to be CO_2) released from limestone and acid could extinguish combustion. Joseph Priestly (1733-1804) recognized that living plants make air "sweet and wholesome"; found that mercuric oxide when heated released a gas which lengthened enclosed animal's survival. Yet all investigators but Black supported the concept of "phlogiston".

Finally, Antoine L Lavoisier (1743-1794), a brilliant and meticulous scientist, through clever experiments with plants, animals and minerals identified three separate and distinct gases: (a) O_2 (respirable portion of the atmosphere); (b) CO_2 (aeriform calcic acid) and (c) N_2 (poisonous or non-respirable portion of the atmosphere). He concluded:

- Respiration affects only the eminently respirable air (O_2); the rest of the atmosphere, the mephitic part (N_2) remains unchanged.
- The calcinations, i.e., heating of solid materials to release gases (i.e., CO_2) or to add gases (i.e., oxidation) to metals in atmospheric air goes on until the eminently respirable air (O_2) contained in the atmosphere is exhausted and combined with the metal. The process will not go on afterwards.
- Animals shut up in confined atmosphere succumb, so soon as they have absorbed or converted the greater part of the respirable portion of the atmosphere (O_2), into aeriform calci acid (CO_2) leaving a remainder (N_2).
- This remainder (N_2 or non-respirable portion of the atmosphere) is the same in calcinations and in respiration, provided that in the latter case, the aeriform calcic acid (CO_2) be removed, and in any case is reconverted into ordinary atmospheric air by adding to it eminently respirable air (O_2).

Thus the theory of phlogiston finally died. Unfortunately, Lavoisier, who was also a tax collector, died prematurely by guillotine during the French Revolution.

ENERGY AND HEAT PRODUCTION

The mystery of heat and energy production was not yet resolved. Combustion and metabolism were not linked. Several investigators [A Crawford, Glasgow (1748-1795); L Spallanzani, Bologna (1729-1799); and HG Magnus (1802-1879)] discovered that venous blood contained more CO_2 and less O_2 than arterial blood, which contained more O_2 and less CO_2. Claude Bernard (1813-1878) found that the temperature of blood leaving organs was higher than that of blood entering the same organs; EFW Pfluger (1829-1910) showed that oxidation occurred in tissues, coined the term respiratory quotient (RQ), and showed that the metabolic needs of tissue were accounted for by the O_2 extracted from capillaries. JR von Mayer (1814-1878) and H Von Helmholtz (1821-1894) fostered the concept of conservation of energy and Max Rubner (1854-1932) meticulously proved the validity of this concept in living dogs.

MECHANICS OF BREATHING AND LUNG VOLUMES

Galen taught and John Mayow confirmed many years later that the lung inflation and deflation followed passively movements of the thorax. Borelli, in 1680, called attention to the air remaining in the lung after complete exhalation (residual air or residual volume). GE Hamburger, in 1727 and 1751, gave a mechanical-mathematical analysis of respiratory movements. Humphrey Davy, in the early 1800s, used H_2 as a tracer gas to calculate what we now call the residual volume.

If it is appropriate to identify Galen and Vesalius as the fathers of anatomy, Harvey as the father of physiology and Lavoisier as the father of chemistry, it is certainly appropriate to identify John Hutchinson as the father of pulmonary function testing.

He presented his treatise "On the content of the lungs and on the respiratory functions, with a view of establishing a precise and easy method of detecting disease by the spirometer" on April 28, 1846, to the Medical-Surgical Society in London.[3] He built and described a water-filled spirometer consisting of a cylinder, closed on one end with attached valving, scales and a water manometer. He described residual air (residual volume), reserve air (expiratory reserve volume), breathing air (tidal volume), complemental air (inspiratory reserve volume) and the vital capacity. He presented many drawings of thoracic and abdominal movements during breathing, and reported the chest circumferences, heights, weights, ages and vital capacities of nearly 2,000 healthy men of various occupations, a few "girls", and 60 diseased patients. His detailed data demonstrated the dependence of vital capacity on gender, age and height, with minimal dependence on weight or chest circumference. Despite his many transthoracic measurements and drawings he was unable to calculate residual air or total lung capacity. He demonstrated the differences in expiratory and inspiratory force in men of different occupations. He made serial observations on patients, some of whom he followed to their death and post-mortem examination. He pointed out that the measurements of vital capacity would be clinically useful to physicians and economically useful to those assuring (insuring) life.

Between 1887 and 1911 nearly a dozen investigators used hydrogen as a tracer to measure residual volume while slightly fewer used O_2 inhalations to dilute O_2 concentrations with or without forced breathing.[4] RV Christie,[4] in 1932, described a detailed method of N_2 dilution with O_2 which was used extensively by Hurtado and colleagues[5] in a large number of healthy and diseased subjects. Christie's method was replaced after 1940 by the widely and currently used N_2 washout technique of Darling and colleagues[6-8] which was found to be more reproducible.

Meanwhile Binger and colleagues and McMichael[4] had introduced satisfactory H_2 equilibration techniques for measuring functional residual capacity, which were quickly replaced in 1949 by the safer helium equilibration method of Meneely and Kaltreider,[9] a method still commonly used.

So-called pneumatometric methods, i.e., dependent on compression and decompression of the lung, were introduced by Pfluger in 1882 to assess total lung capacity. However, these methods were poorly reproducible.[4] The body plethysmographic technique with panting maneuvers, as developed and explained by DuBois and colleagues in 1956,[10] is now the only such technique relying on compression and decompression of thoracic gas volume.

CARBON MONOXIDE (CO) TRANSFER IN THE LUNG

Marie and August Krogh[11] first developed the brief breath-holding technique, which required both early and late expired samples, to measure the transfer of CO in the lung. This was further simplified and developed by Forster, Ogilvie and their colleagues by adding a tracer gas. Their slightly modified procedure is now currently and extensively used.[12-14] Although H_2 was first used as the tracer gas it was soon replaced by helium, then later by neon, and later by methane, the latter because the exhaled alveolar gas could be continually analyzed for both CO and methane. Meanwhile, Filley and colleagues[15] developed the exercise "steady state method" for assessing CO uptake, a procedure now rarely used due to the simplicity and reproducibility of the single breath test.

BLOOD O_2 AND CO_2 CONTENTS AND TRANSPORT

Hoppe-Seyler Felix (1825-1895) isolated and obtained crystallized hemoglobin in 1882 and described many attributes of hemoglobin and related compounds. Paul Bert (1833-1886), in addition to his high-altitude work showing that O_2 pressure is critical for existence whereas barometric pressure is not critical, published the first oxyhemoglobin dissociation curve in 1872. Christian Bohr (1855-1911) further developed the S-shaped oxyhemoglobin curve and is credited with graphically demonstrating that blood CO_2 contents are influenced by O_2 contents (and vice versa). In the earlier 20th century, a great number of investigators (e.g., Joseph Barcroft, J Christiansen, Julius Comroe, Andre Cournand, Bruce Dill, Walter Fenn, JS Haldane, JH Hasselbalch, Lawrence Y Henderson, Marie and August Krogh, Herman Rahn, Richard Riley, FWJ Roughton and Donald Van Slyke) added to knowledge regarding blood O_2 and CO_2 content and transport within the human body at rest and during exercise.

REFERENCES

1. Perkins JF Jr. Historical development of respiratory physiology. In: WO Fenn, H Rahn (Eds). Handbook of Physiology. Washington DC: American Physiological Society; 1964.
2. The Holy Bible, New Revised Standard Version. Iowa Falls, Iowa: World Bible Publishers; 1989.
3. Hutchinson J. On the capacity of the lungs and on the respiratory functions, with the view of establishing a precise and easy method of detecting disease by the spirometer. *Medical-Chirurgical Transactions (London).* 1846;29:137-252.
4. Christie RV. The lung volume and its subdivisions. *J Clin Invest.* 1932;11:1099-118.
5. Hurtado A, Boller C. Studies of total pulmonary capacity and its subdivisions. Normal, absolute, and relative values. *J Clin Invest.* 1933;12:793-806.
6. Darling RC, Cournand A, Mansfield JS, et al. Studies on the intrapulmonary mixture of gases. Nitrogen elimination from blood and body tissues during high oxygen breathing. *J Clin Invest.* 1940;19:591-7.
7. Cournand A, Darling RC, Mansfield JS, et al. Studies on the intrapulmonary mixture of gases. Analysis of the rebreathing method (closed circuit) for measuring residual air. *J Clin Invest.* 1940;19:599-608.

8. Darling RC, Cournand A, Richards DW Jr. Studies on the intrapulmonary mixture of gases. An open circuit method for measuring residual air. *J Clin Invest.* 1940;19:609-18.

9. Meneely GR, Kaltreider NL. The volume of the lung determined by helium dilution. Description of the method and comparison with other procedures. *J Clin Invest.* 1949;28:129-39.

10. DuBois AB, Botelho SY, Bedell GN, et al. A rapid plethysmographic method for measuring thoracic gas volume: A comparison with nitrogen washout method for measuring functional residual capacity in normal subjects. *J Clin Invest.* 1956;35:322-6.

11. Krogh M. Diffusion of gases through the lungs of man. *J Physiol.* 1915;49:271-300.

12. Forster RE, Fowler WS, Bates DV, et al. The absorption of carbon monoxide by the lungs during breathholding. *J Clin Invest.* 1954;33:1125-45.

13. Forster RE, Cohn JE, Briscoe WA, et al. A modification of the Krogh carbon monoxide breath holding technique for estimating the diffusing capacity of the lung: a comparison with three other methods. *J Clin Invest.* 1955;34:1417-26.

14. Ogilvie CM, Forster RE, Blakemore WS, et al. A standardized breath holding technique for the clinical measurement of the diffusing capacity of the lung for carbon monoxide. *J Clin Invest.* 1957;36:1-17.

15. Filley GF, MacIntosh DJ, Wright GW. Carbon monoxide uptake and pulmonary diffusing capacity in normal subjects at rest and during exercise. *J Clin Invest.* 1954;33:530-9.

2 Structure and Function

INTRODUCTION

We will consider some of the structures of the normal thoracic cage and its contents so that we can better understand lung function in health and disease. History, physical examination and a variety of other radiological techniques give us differing perspectives regarding lung health. Safe and non-invasive techniques and procedures in the pulmonary function laboratory give us low cost, immediate and useful information regarding the ability or inability of the individual to adequately ventilate the airspaces and transfer O_2 and CO_2 between the airspaces and the pulmonary capillaries.

Lung diseases can be considered: obstructive (gas cannot quickly get out from the airspaces back to the atmosphere), restrictive (the lung is reduced in size), and/or vascular (transfer of O_2 and CO_2 between the airspaces and the pulmonary capillaries is inhibited by reduction in pulmonary capillary blood volume or flow or barriers between the airspaces and the capillaries). Examples: (a) purely obstructive disease are uncomplicated asthma or chronic bronchitis; (b) purely restrictive are pleural effusion, pneumothorax or extreme obesity; (c) purely vascular are pulmonary vasculopathy associated with idiopathic pulmonary hypertension; (d) both obstructive and restrictive are some pneumoconiosis and sarcoidosis; (e) both obstructive and vascular are emphysema; (f) both restrictive and vascular are interstitial lung diseases or pulmonary emboli with infarction and (g) combined obstructive, restrictive and vascular are heart failure with pulmonary edema. How can the laboratory help identify these disorders? How can we monitor their progression or regression over time or with therapy?

THE THORACIC "CAGE"

The human body is a marvelous structure and the thorax enclosing the lungs, heart, diaphragm and major blood vessels is no exception. The bony thorax includes the thoracic spine, 12 paired ribs and sternum. The upper 6 pairs of ribs directly articulate with the sternum, whereas the 7th through 10th pair connect to the sternum through cartilage and the last 2 pairs of ribs connect to the sternum only through soft tissue. During quiet inspiration, the scalene and sternocleidomastoid muscles can move the first rib up and outward; the intercostal muscles move the 2nd through 6th ribs up and outward something like the handle of a bucket. The 7th through 10th ribs tend to move laterally outward during inspiration, increasing the lateral thoracic diameter and reducing the anteroposterior diameter of the thorax. The muscles of the diaphragm originate from the inferior portions of the thoracic cage, including the costal margins and xiphoid process of the sternum. The muscle fibers converge on the central tendon of the diaphragm. With quiet inspiration, the central tendon and the diaphragm move abdominally a centimeter or so, increasing the volume and decreasing the pressure within the thoracic cage while increasing the pressure within the abdomen. With low ventilatory requirements, expiration is primarily passive due to the inherent elastic recoil properties of the lung.

With heavy exercise, ventilatory requirements can increase more than tenfold, accomplished both by increasing the volume of each breath 4–6 times and the frequency of breathing 2–3 times. When ventilatory requirements increase, contractions of the pectoralis major and minor and latissimus dorsi add to the inspiratory movements of the upper thorax. In addition, the diaphragm contraction and movement increases manyfold during inspiration and the anterior abdominal muscles contract more forcefully during expiration to force the diaphragm upward.

The thorax also contains many other structures, such as the esophagus, lymphatics, nerves, fat, cartilage, bones and musculature, but our major emphasis in understanding pulmonary function relates to the lungs and heart and the thoracic cage. Ventilation and perfusion are also influenced by structures outside the thorax, including the upper airways, the central nervous, endocrine and immunologic systems, and most importantly by the metabolism of the rest of the body which utilizes oxygen (O_2) and returns carbon dioxide (CO_2) to the lungs through the vascular system. The lung then extracts O_2 from the atmosphere in quantities necessary to maintain good oxygen saturation in the systemic arterial blood and returns CO_2 to the atmosphere in appropriate quantities so that the ratio of CO_2 to bicarbonate (HCO_3^-) and concentration of hydrogen ion [H^+] in the periphery are maintained within a narrow range.

VOLUMES AND CAPACITIES OF THE LUNG

The lung volume is identified as total lung capacity (TLC) when the lung is fully inflated in the thorax. With complete exhalation, the lung volume is identified as residual volume (RV). The difference between the TLC and the RV is the vital capacity (VC), i.e., the amount of inhaled volume from RV to TLC or exhaled volume from TLC to RV. The volume of air (or gas) during each breath is the tidal volume (VT). The volume which can be further inhaled from the inspiratory end of VT breathing is identified as the inspiratory reserve volume; the amount that can be further exhaled from the expiratory end of VT breathing is the expiratory reserve volume (ERV). This state at the end of quiet exhalation is considered the resting position of the lung and differs considerably from the position and volume of the lungs seen on either full inspiratory or full expiratory chest radiographs. By tradition, when any volumes are combined, they are identified as capacities. An important capacity is the functional residual capacity (FRC), which is the combination of the ERV and the RV. Another is the inspiratory capacity (IC) which is the combination of VT and IRV. As can be seen in figures 2-1 and 2-2, the VC = IRV +TV + ERV, or VC = ERV + IC; TLC = VC +

Normal lung volumes and capacities

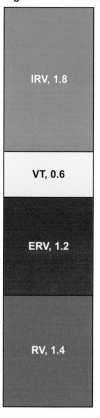

Figure 2-1 The volumes of the lung displayed vertically with residual volume (RV) below and inspiratory reserve volume (IRV) above. Expiratory reserve volume (ERV) and RV equal functional residual capacity (FRC). IRV and tidal volume (VT) equal inspratory capacity (IC). IRV, VT and ERV = vital capacity (VC), as do IC and FRC. All volumes together equal total lung capacity (TLC). These are approximate values for a normal 25-year-old Latin male 170 cm tall. Although spirometirc values are often displayed this way this is really upside down compared to the anatomy of a standing subject.[1]

RV, or TLC = IC + FRC, or TLC = IRV + TV + ERV + RV. Every individual measuring or interpreting pulmonary function tests should be familiar with these relationships.

The VC is predominantly dependent on age, height, and gender, and to a variable way on ethnicity. The predicted values of VC derived from approximately 5,000 NHANES-3 never-smoking adults are shown in figure 2-3. Note that for the same age and height, men have significantly larger VC than women of the same age and height. Although there are minimal differences between the Latin and white adults of the same gender, black men and women have significantly lower VC than their white and Latin counterparts of the same heights.

The proportions and ratios of the lung volumes change with nutritional status, but the VC and TLC are relatively unaffected (Figure 2-4) unless obesity is severe.

Normal lung volumes and capacities

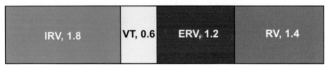

Figure 2-2 The same lung volumes and symbols as displayed in Figure 2-1 from RV on the right to TLC on the left. In this case, the head of the supine subject is on the right, not the left.

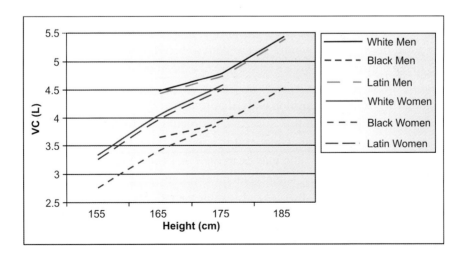

Figure 2-3 Mean vital capacity (VC) values for 40-year-old never-smoking men and women showing dependency on height, gender and ethnicity. Ten years younger subjects would have larger VC's and 10 years older subjects would have smaller VC's.[1]

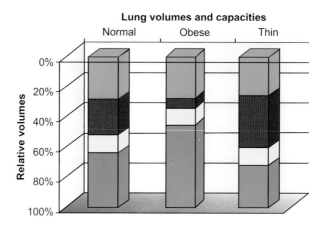

Figure 2-4 Lung volumes and capacities as modified by nutritional status. In these depictions, the subjects are upright: the gray extends to the superior end of the thorax and the blue extends to the inferior end of the thorax. Lung volumes are as follows: blue = residual volume (RV), red = expiratory reserve volume (ERV), yellow = tidal volume (TV) and green = inspiratory reserve volume (IRV). Lung capacities are: red plus blue = functional residual capacity (FRC), yellow plus green = inspiratory capacity (IC) and red plus yellow plus green = vital capacity (VC) and blue plus red plus yellow plus green = total lung capacity (TLC). The position of the diaphragm is as follows: in the yellow with quiet breathing, between the yellow and the green at quiet end-inspiration, between the red and yellow at quiet end-expiration, below the green at full inspiration, and between the blue and red at full expiration.

During resting breathing, when tidal volume is low, the diaphragm moves in the yellow zone, between the red and green. With a forced inhalation, the diaphragm moves to the bottom of the green; with a forced exhalation it moves to between the red and the blue. With obesity, especially when involving the chest and abdomen, the resting end-expiratory position of the diaphragm is elevated between the yellow and the red (mid panel); in thin subjects, the resting end-expiratory position of the diaphragm between the yellow and the red is much lower (right panel). In obesity, the resting IC/ERV ratio may be as high as 4:1 to 10:1, or even more. Thus, from a resting state, the obese subject can inhale deeply and move the diaphragm a significant distance caudad, but can only exhale a small expiratory reserve volume, moving the diaphragm a short distance cephalad. In a thin individual, the IC/ERV ratio is closer to 1:1, the IC tends to be decreased and the ERV increased (right panel). From a resting state the thin individual can exhale deeply and move the diaphragm a large distance cephalad, but with inhalation, the inspiratory reserve volume is less than in the less thin, and the diaphragm moves a relatively short distance caudad. With extreme overnutrition and undernutrition there are small changes in VC.

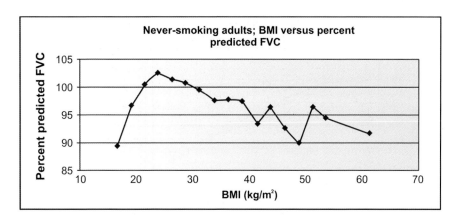

Figure 2-5 Relatively small changes in forced vital capacity (FVC) as body mass index (BMI) changes over a very wide range. Data are from over 5,000 NHANES-3 never-smoking adults of three ethnicities.[1]

In the NHANES-3 population of never-smokers, figure 2-5 shows the relationship between actual and predicted VC measures in 5,000 never-smokers, arranged by body mass index (BMI). Note that the ratio of actual to predicted VC values, which are based on height, age, gender and ethnicity, but not weight, are below 100% in those few subjects with the lowest BMI, slightly above 100% for the large number of subjects with BMI's from 20 to 30 group, and well below 100% as BMI increases to 40 or above.

The lung volumes and capacities also change in never-smoking adults with aging, independent of any disease process. Cross-sectional studies are not ideal for identifying changes with normal aging, but offer some insight. In the NHANES-3 study, e.g., the height of never-smoking participants in each portion, whether black, Latin or white, or men or women, decreased, on average, slightly less than 1.0 cm per decade from the mid-fourth to mid-eighth decade (Figures 2-6 and 2-7). This could minimally be due to changes in nutrition status of each population over these 5 decades, but more likely relates to some "settling" of the spine, especially in those over age 50 years, relating to decreasing bone density. Meanwhile, the VC changed considerably more than height. Ethnicity does not seem to be a factor in these aging changes. Regardless of the absolute change in height assumed for a given individual, the volume shifts are striking.

Published series which combine both flow and complete lung volume equations are much less common than those using only spirometry. As one can see, the mean heights in the never-smoking NHANES-3 population decline as age increases by and after the mid-fifth decades. This may be partly due to differences in nutrition between 1915 and 1995, but is also due to shortening of the spine with increasing age, both

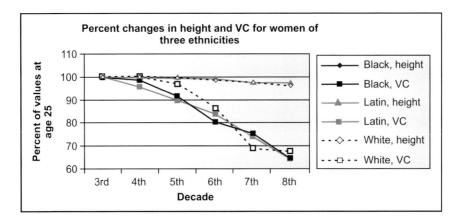

Figure 2-6 Mean height and VC in NHANES-3 women of three ethnicities by mid-decade as compared to mean values at age 25 years (3rd decade).[1]

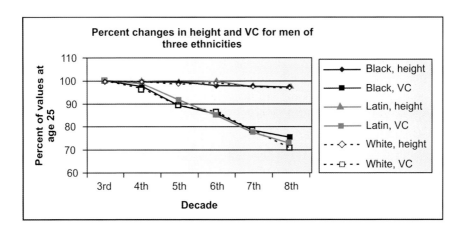

Figure 2-7 Mean height and VC in NHANES-3 men of three ethnicities by mid-decade as compared to mean values at age 25 years (3rd decade).[1]

in men and women. The results of calculating TLC and VC, with the difference as RV, using four pairs of frequently used reference[2-5] equations for populations at ages 35 and 75 for given heights are shown in table 2-1. Mean values of VC, RV and TLC using reference equations of ERS, Cotes, Crapo and Gutierrez[2-5] show their relative sizes expected with aging for a typical never-smoking man and typical never-smoking woman. The decreases of VC/TLC and increases of RV/TLC and especially RV/VC with aging are quite dramatic in both men and women. The increases in RV and decreases in VC over time in women and men of all three ethnicities must in part be due to decreases in elastic recoil of the lung (Figures 2-8 and 2-9 and Table 2-1)

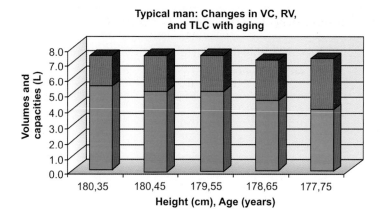

Figure 2-8 Changes in VC (green), RV (red) and TLC (red and green together) in a given normal man 180 cm tall at age 35, presuming a 1 cm reduction in height each decade from ages 45 to 75 years.

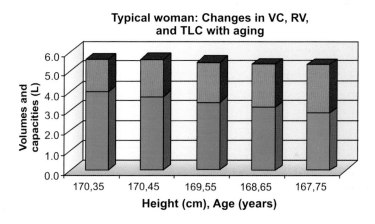

Figure 2-9 Changes in VC (green), RV (red) and TLC (red and green together) in a given normal woman 170 cm tall at age 35, presuming a 1 cm reduction in height each decade from ages 45 to 75 years.

AIRWAYS

Structure

Gases move in and out of the lung in airways, where bulk flow predominates (all gases move in the same direction) and in air spaces, where diffusion predominates (and O_2 and CO_2 can move in opposite directions). During inhalation, the intrathoracic

Table 2-1	Changes in Total Lung Capacity (TLC), Vital Capacity (VC) and Residual Volume (RV) and Their Ratios from Age 35 to 75 years in Men or Women, Assuming that Height is Likely to Decrease by 0, 2, and 3 cm Over a 40 year Period[1-5]		
	No change	**2 cm decrease**	**3 cm decrease**
Men	180 cm, 35 yrs 180 cm, 75 yrs	178 cm, 75 yrs	177 cm, 75 yrs
TLC, L	7.32 7.37	7.20	7.12
VC, L	5.41 4.47	4.35	4.29
RV, L	1.91 2.89	2.85	2.83
RV/TLC	0.26 0.39	0.40	0.40
VC/TLC	0.74 0.61	0.60	0.60
RV/VC	0.35 0.65	0.66	0.66
Women	170 cm, 35 yrs 170 cm, 75 yrs	168 cm, 75 yrs	167 cm, 75 yrs
TLC, L	5.59 5.50	5.37	5.31
VC, L	3.97 3.05	2.96	2.91
RV, L	1.63 2.45	2.41	2.40
RV/TLC	0.29 0.45	0.45	0.45
VC/TLC	0.71 0.55	0.55	0.55
RV/VC	0.41 0.80	0.81	0.82

pressure is less than atmospheric, causing inward bulk flow. During exhalation, the intrathoracic pressure is necessarily more positive than atmospheric, causing outward bulk flow.

Traveling inward, the airways begin at the mouth and nose and continue through the pharynx and larynx and external trachea before finally reaching and entering the thoracic cage. The trachea then bifurcates near the heart into a major bronchus for each side of the body (Figure 2-10).[6] Thereafter, each airway (bronchus) bifurcates somewhat irregularly a few times into one of five lobes and 18 segments and then systematically bifurcates again and again until the airways become terminal bronchioles. The airway branching pattern within each segment is invariably bifurcating, with the major and larger of the two daughters deviating slightly from the direction of the parent and the minor daughter and smaller of the two daughters deviating away from the direction of the parent.[6] If we count the bifurcation of the trachea to major bronchi as generation "one", the number of bifurcations or generations to reach the terminal bronchiole varies from as few as 7 or 8 to as many as 22 or 23. Generally, the terminal bronchioles of lower numbered generations are located more centrally and those of higher numbered generations more peripherally.

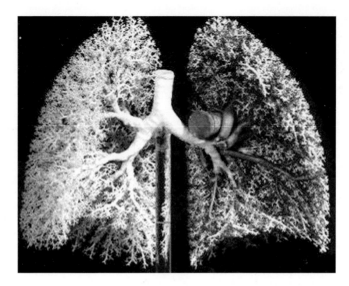

Figure 2-10 Cast of the larger human airways showing the pattern of irregular dichotomy in the lobar volumes with the larger daughter usually continuing more directly and the smaller daughter deviating.[6]

Weibel[6] clearly recognized that the airways often branched irregularly (Figure 2-11), but that knowledge is frequently ignored by others as his famous diagram depicting regular dichotomy (Figure 2-12) rather than irregular dichotomy is almost invariably reproduced in other publications.

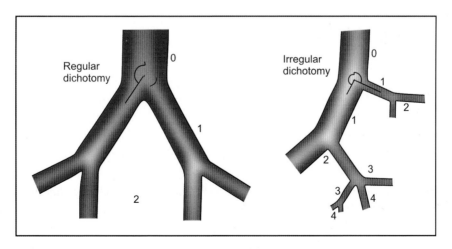

Figure 2-11 A diagram of Weibel showing regular dichotomy as well as irregular branching of airways.[6]

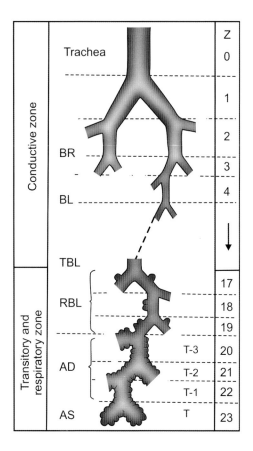

Figure 2-12 Famous and frequently copied diagram of Weibel showing number of generations and regular dichotomy of airways and airspaces of the human lung. In his monograph Weibel emphasized that the branching of airways was commonly irregular dichotomy rather than regular dichotomy depicted in this figure.[6]

The total volume of the airways in the average adult is remarkably small, less than 120 mL or so at complete exhalation and 240 mL or so at complete inhalation. No significant gas exchange occurs in the airways. These "freeways" allow bulk flow only in one direction at a time and are highly efficient parts of a two-way "in and out" transport system. If we calculate 2 to the 15th power (the average number of bifurcations), the number of terminal bronchioles (and acini) equals approximately 30,000, one less generation than that suggested by Weibel.[6] As detailed later, his description of three generations of respiratory bronchioles is reasonable but Weibel's assumption of three bifurcating generations of alveolar ducts overestimates their individual length and underestimates their number. As a consequence, the complexity of the branching pattern of the airspaces is underestimated and the distances from the terminal bronchioles in the acinus to the airspace capillaries are overestimated by his model.

Flow

Bulk air flow requires differences in pressure, with bulk flow of air (or gases) during ventilation always moving from higher to lower pressures until the pressures equalize. Figure 2-13 demonstrates the changes in bulk expiratory volume (and flows) in typical never-smoking women from age 25 to 75. Note that with increasing age, the VC at 8 seconds gradually decreases while the volumes at 1, 2 and 3 seconds decrease slightly more (the red, orange, olive, green and blue are a little more distant from the black line at these times).

Figures 2-14 to 2-17 show how different measurements of expiratory flow are influenced by differing degrees of airway obstruction which may be due to the aging process or disease. The legends are explanatory and show some of the theoretical disadvantages of the $FEF_{25-75\%}$ measurements and the advantages of the FEV_1/FVC and the FEV_3/FVC or $1-FEV_3/FVC$. Not shown is the high inherent variability of the $FEF_{25-75\%}$ (and the $FEF_{25\%}$, $FEF_{50\%}$, $FEF_{75\%}$) measurements and the low inherent variability of the FEV_1/FVC and FEV_3/FVC measurements in a sample population of any given age, gender, ethnicity or height.

AIRSPACES

Earlier Findings

In 1832,[7] Laennec wrote of emphysema, "To enable us to have a correct notion of this disease, we must inflate the affected lungs and dry them. If they are then cut

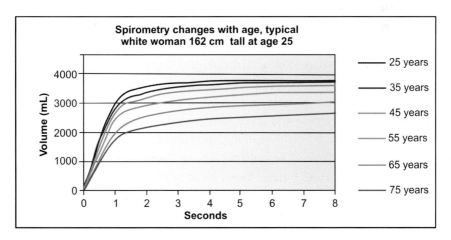

Figure 2-13 Changes in timed lung volumes with aging in a never-smoking white woman who was 162 cm tall at age 25 years.[1]

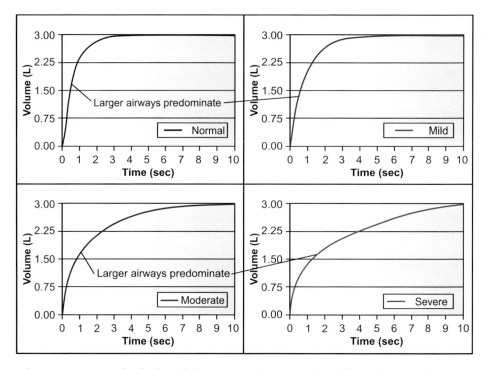

Figure 2-14 Four individuals with the same vital capacity but differing degrees of airway obstruction. The arrows point to the portions of the tracings where flow is dominantly affected by the larger airways, i.e., in the first second or so, when volume changes the fastest. This tendency is true regardless of the degree of airway obstruction.[1]

into slices with a fine instrument, we perceive at once that the air cells are almost always more dilated than they appear externally." How incredibly perceptive! Over a hundred years later, the anatomy, physiology, and pathology of the human lungs became much clearer when Gough and Wentworth[8] began mounting thin slices of the fixed lung so that its mesoanatomy and pathology could be examined, and Weibel and colleagues[6] perfected better techniques for inflating and fixing the post-mortem lung through the trachea. These techniques allowed under relatively minor magnification, better understanding of airway and acinar anatomy, physiology and pathology.[9]

Weibel increased understanding of the anatomy of the airways and airspaces by using morphometric counting techniques, i.e., by counting under the microscope on thin sections of normal human fixed, inflated and sectioned lung each time and distance when superimposed straight lines intersected tissue. He tested his hypothesis regarding numbers and shapes of airspaces by correctly ascertaining the size, number and shape of beans and peas which had been fixed in gelatin, sectioned and morphometrically examined microscopically. Because this approach confirmed

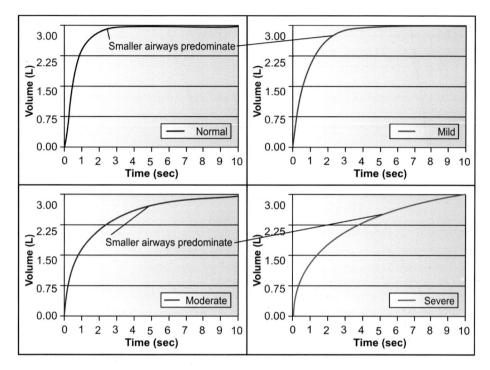

Figure 2-15 Four individuals with the same vital capacity but differing degrees of airway obstruction. The arrows point to the portions of the tracings where flow is dominantly affected by the smaller airways and the airspaces which empty later, i.e., in the later seconds, when volume changes the slowest or least. This tendency is true regardless of the degree of airway obstruction.[1]

his hypothesis, he used his formulas and counting techniques on thin slices of lung to determine and report his findings regarding the shape, sizes and numbers of alveolar ducts, sacs and alveoli. Figure 2-12 is correct for airways but not for airspaces.

Later Findings

We took a different approach to the problem of studying the mesoanatomy of the acinus which altered our knowledge of the acinar airspaces. We inflated, fixed and sliced nearly 200 consecutive 0.020 mm sections of a small portion of the lung of a young never-smoking woman who had died suddenly in an accident. Images of these serial sections were magnified and projected in a darkened room unto thin circles of semi-rigid foam a centimeter thick and 150 cm in diameter. The tissue outlines were carefully traced, with the open spaces equivalent to lumens of the airspaces and airways. These open spaces were then cut out and discarded. By temporarily

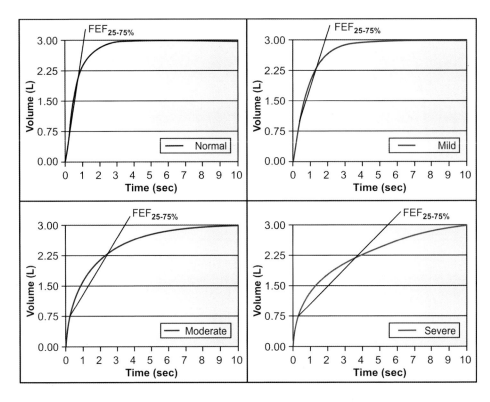

Figure 2-16 The same four individuals with the same vital capacity but differing degrees of airway obstruction. The diagonal lines are tangents. Each tangent connects the volume and time at 25% of FVC with volume and time at 75% of FVC. Each is the $FEF_{25-75\%}$, the mean flow between these points. Note that in this normal, the $FEF_{25-75\%}$ is complete before the FEV_1, with mild obstruction is complete very near the FEV_1, with moderate obstruction at about the FEV_2, and with severe obstruction at about FEV_4. Thus each $FEF_{25-75\%}$ value is time dependent and measures different portions of the expiratory flow.[1]

retaining the prior section on the wall, it was not difficult to find and project, and trace the next section. Eight to ten complete sections were then glued together and the 150 cm circles cut into quadrants.[10] A terminal bronchiole, three generations of respiratory bronchioles were identified and the airspaces evaluated. The shapes and branching patterns of the airspaces were unexpected but were carefully examined in all directions, counted, color coded, numbered, and measured in three directions. By using a combination of numbers and colors and a defined logic we were able to define the branching pattern and estimate the numbers, sizes and shapes of alveolar ducts, alveolar sacs and alveoli. An alveolar sac is defined as the last generation of

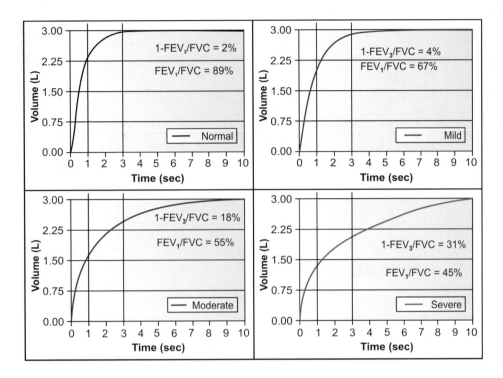

Figure 2-17 The same four individuals with measurements of FEV_1/FVC and $1-FEV_3/FVC$. The FEV_1/FVC is the fraction (or percentage) of FVC exhaled in the first second; the $1-FEV_3/FVC$ is the fraction (or percentage) of FVC exhaled after 3 seconds. The $1-FEV_3/FVC$ (easily calculated from $FVC-FEV_3/FVC$) is a measurement of late flow, i.e., invariably from the smaller airways and slower emptying airspaces. Proportionally, it may change equally, less or even more than the FEV_1/FVC as airway obstruction increases.[1]

alveolar duct before terminating solely in alveoli. Sacs most commonly divided into two alveoli, but occasionally into as many as eight alveoli (Figure 2-18).

Each terminal bronchiole enters a single acinus, a portion of which is shown diagrammatically in figure 2-18. Each terminal bronchiole, the entrance and exit for air of the approximately spherical acinus, branches dichotomously three times, into three generations of *respiratory* bronchioles. These generations of bronchioles are named "respiratory" because they have a few, but increasing number of alveoli and sacs on their lateral surfaces as the generation number increases. The respiratory bronchioles allow both bulk flow (ventilation) to the alveolar ducts and gas exchange (diffusion) to their relatively few lateral alveoli. There are three generations of

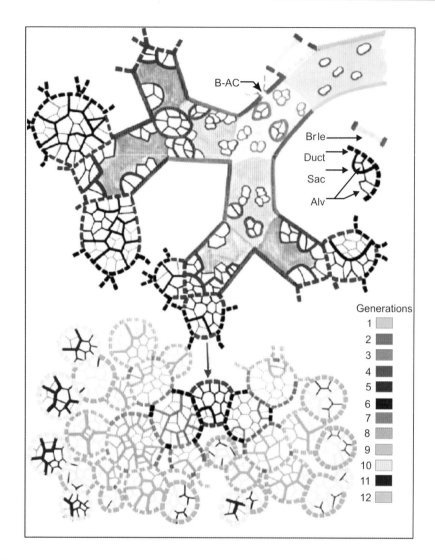

Figure 2-18 A model of a portion of a human acinus with a different color for each generation, counting the terminal bronchiole entering and defining the acinus as generation 1. It is difficult to analyze, understand and portray a three-dimensional structure in two dimensions, either on a slide under the microscope or on a page. The three generations of respiratory bronchioles (2, 3, and 4) have mostly lateral solid walls but are increasingly defined by airspaces (alveoli and sacs) as they enter the center of the acinus. The respiratory bronchioles branch into ducts, each of which branches directly and immediately into more ducts, sacs and alveoli. The ducts are present in generations 5–11, sacs in generations 3–12 and alveoli in generations 3–13. Each alveolar duct tended to be ovoid or spherical before branching.[10]

respiratory bronchioles, thus there are eight third generation respiratory bronchioles in the typical acinus (2 × 2 × 2 = 8). Branching continues distally, but the pattern of branching changes markedly. The third generation or final respiratory bronchioles branch completely into airspaces (ducts, sacs and alveoli). Each respiratory bronchiole is approximately 1 mm in length and 0.5 mm in diameter. By the third generation, respiratory bronchioles are long enough to efficiently reach the center of the acinus.

For many decades, since anatomists, pathologists and physiologists looked at two-dimensional human lung sections under the microscope, the alveolar ducts were compared to hallways, with alveolar sacs and alveoli lining their sides. In two-dimensions, this is the appearance of many alveolar ducts. This appearance is not illogical, but was found to be incorrect by examining a three dimensional model.[11] Considering the number of alveoli in an acinus, Weibel and others logically assumed that there were three generations of bifurcating "hall-like" alveolar ducts to accommodate the number of alveoli they counted. However, in our three-dimensional reconstruction of a normal acinus (enlarged over 300 times in each dimension) this pattern was never seen. Rather, alveolar ducts were ovoid or spherical and branched profusely into several daughters, i.e., into other alveolar ducts plus alveolar sacs and alveoli. Since the alveolar ducts were surfaced predominantly with airspaces, not tissue, their shapes, sizes and dimensions could not be expected to be correctly ascertained from two-dimensional morphometric analyses, i.e., the counting of tissue crossings of two-dimensional thin sections. Thus, the number, shapes and sizes of alveolar ducts of human lung could not be determined from these techniques. In the reconstructed three-dimensional acinus, there were up to six to eight generations of alveolar ducts found coming from each third generation respiratory bronchiole.[12]

The respiratory bronchioles and first three generations of alveolar ducts tend to be similar in diameter of about 500 microns, but further alveolar duct lengths then immediately and progressively decreased going peripherally. For these later generations the ducts became ovoid or spherical as both their diameters and lengths declined from 500–600 microns to 200–250 microns. The dimensions and numbers are given in table 2-2 and figure 2-19.[12]

The alveoli are diverse in shape, but are generally shaped like deep bowls or deep saucers. They can be characterized as portions of spheroids, cylindroids, ellipsoids or truncated cones, generally sharing common walls with other alveoli. The average diameter of a single alveolus approximates 200 microns, their average surface area approximates 0.10 mm^2, and their average volume approximates 0.0040 mm^3. Alveoli occupy approximately half of the total acinar volume. At a TLC of 5.5 L, the average acinar volume and diameter approximate 200 mm^3 and 7.2 mm. At an RV

Table 2-2	Approximate Numbers and Sizes of Respiratory Bronchioles, Ducts, Sacs and Alveoli in a Typical Human Adult Acinus[12]			
Name of airspace	Generation number	Total number	Length (mm)	Diameter (mm)
Respiratory bronchioles	1	2	1.0	0.5
Respiratory bronchioles	2	4	0.98	0.5
Respiratory bronchioles	3	8	0.95	0.5
Total RB		14		
Alveolar ducts	4	19	0.61	0.54
Alveolar ducts	5	45	0.55	0.49
Alveolar ducts	6	108	0.49	0.45
Alveolar ducts	7	254	0.44	0.40
Alveolar ducts	8	374	0.38	0.36
Alveolar ducts	9	366	0.32	0.31
Alveolar ducts	10	146	0.26	0.26
Alveolar ducts	11	58	0.21	0.22
Total alveolar ducts		1370		
Total sacs	3 to 12	2700 to 4200	0.2	0.25
Total alveoli	2 to 13	9500 to 14700	0.2	0.2

of 1.6 L the average acinar volume and diameter approximate 58 mm^3 and 4.8 mm. With inflation of the lung from RV, the alveoli tend to unfold so that acinar surface area is relatively unchanged. Thus, an acinar volume can increase over three times while the acinar diameter increases only by one-half. Considering that there are large numbers of ducts, sacs and tissue and blood within the acinus, the gas within the alveoli occupies approximately half of the acinar volume.

It was challenging to try to understand why our findings in the normal acinus differed so much from those of Weibel's model (Figure 2-12). In evaluating this perplexing issue, we eventually realized that there was the following fallacy in using the counting principle in the lung airspaces.[11] Briefly, two dimensional sections alone cannot distinguish and define the shape and size of an alveolar duct as it can define peas and beans, since alveolar duct "walls" are *not* all tissue (or bark). Rather, the "walls" predominantly consist of their daughter ducts, sacs and airspaces which do not have tissue separating each generation. The marked undercounting of the alveolar ducts and visualization that a single duct, before branching, may be relatively long and narrow on thin sections, was inherent in the Weibel model of airspaces. The Weibel model of the acinus had three bifurcating generations of respiratory bronchioles (which do have predominantly tissue walls and can be correctly counted and measured by his techniques). The Weibel model then required only three generations of long, bifurcating alveolar ducts to accommodate the correctly counted number of alveoli.

This difference in anatomy using the Weibel morphometric model and our three-dimensional reconstruction is important functionally (Figures 2-19 and 2-20). The three-dimensional reconstruction model allows for much shorter diffusion distances and a marked increase in diffusion efficiency of O_2 and CO_2 in the airspaces than the Weibel model. This diffusion efficiency is totally independent of what time it takes for diffusion between the epithelial surface and endothelial surface of the capillary lumen and hemoglobin-containing red cells. The differences between the cross-sectional area, surface area and distance for diffusion of gases as calculated from the Weibel model which has three generations of bifurcating alveolar ducts and the three-dimensional reconstruction which has six to eight generations of shorter branching alveolar ducts is noted on a semilogarithmic plot in figure 2-20. The differences between the models in cross-sectional and surface areas are striking.[12] The three-dimensional reconstruction discloses a much shorter distance for gaseous diffusion and more rapid and efficient exchange of O_2 and CO_2 within the acinus than the Weibel model. Paiva et al.[13] confirmed the validity of the reconstruction model when he found that measurements of gaseous diffusion in the human lung fit the reconstruction model very well.

This pattern found in the three-dimensional reconstruction is ideal for the concurrent diffusion of CO_2 and O_2 within an acinus. Compared to the Weibel model, which has only three generations of long bifurcating ducts, the distances for diffusion and faster O_2 and CO_2 exchange are better in the reconstruction model. If one characterizes the volume and shape of the airways and intra-acinar airspaces from the trachea to the alveolar surfaces, the model only minimally resembles a trumpet-like shape. Instead, it resembles the shape of a giant thumb-tack, terminating with an explosion of surface area over a very short distance. Perhaps a real trumpet of average size without tubing or valves (simulating all the airways) placed on a red-painted half of a tennis court (simulating a 10 micron thick surface of blood in the pulmonary capillaries) would be an appropriate large image to contemplate. What a small volume needs to be ventilated through the horn to reach the very large surface of blood! It is appropriate to note that the N_2, O_2, CO_2 and H_2O are moved by bulk flow (ventilation) in and out of the horn together to the center of the acinus but the O_2 and CO_2 move quickly in opposite directions by partial pressure-driven gaseous diffusion (not ventilation) to the capillary alveolar surface and then by further diffusion predominantly in and out of the capillary hemoglobin.

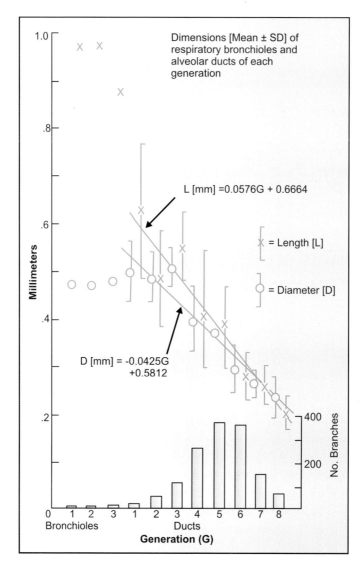

Figure 2-19 The lengths and diameters of the airways (bronchioles) and alveolar ducts found in the reconstruction of a portion of a human acinus. The lengths of the respiratory bronchioles are twice their diameters. By the second generation of alveolar ducts (sixth generation if we count the terminal bronchiole entering the acinus as first generation) and progressing distally, the lengths and diameters of the ducts are nearly equal.[12]

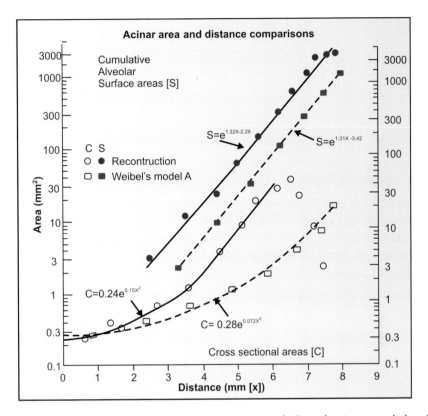

Figure 2-20 Comparison of the airspaces' cross-sectional (C = clear) area and alveolar capillary surface areas (S = solid) within the human acinus using the Weibel model (squares) and the three-dimensional reconstruction model (circles). The Y-axis is a logarithmic scale so that these differences in cross-sectional area and alveolar (capillary) surface area between the two models are really very large. The "x" in the formula is distance in mm. The efficiency of gas exchange is considerably better in the reconstruction since the distances for diffusion of CO_2 and O_2 within the acinus are considerably less in the reconstruction.[12]

Alveoli and acini vary in size and are dependent on the phase of the ventilatory cycle and the effect of gravity. Glazier and colleagues[14] innovatively studied alveolar sizes in anesthetized dogs in head up and head down positions with their intact lungs frozen at full inspiration and expiration. They verified that alveolar size was dependent both on the ventilatory cycle and the position of the lung in relation to gravity (Figure 2-21). Recall that with breathing, volume increases and decreases many times more than diameter of airspace does. At full exhalation, whether frozen in the head up or head down position, the inferior dependent airspaces were smaller, even atelectatic, whereas superior higher airspaces were not as small. At

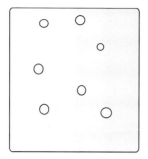 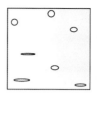

Figure 2-21 Alveolar shape and size at full inspiration or total lung capacity (left) and full expiration or residual volume (right) at the apex (top) and base (bottom) of the lung in the upright position. At full inspiration the airspaces are more spherical. At full expiration, especially inferiorly, the airspaces are compressed and tend to become disc-like or folded. Recall that the volume of a sphere or cube is really related to the cube of its diameter while in the diagram, the area of a circle or rectangle is related to the square of its diameter.

full inhalation, inferior and superior airspaces were more equal in size. Thus, the uppermost alveoli change less in volume with a given ventilation (i.e., ventilated less) while the lowermost alveoli change more in volume with the same ventilation (i.e., ventilated more). Translating these findings to upright humans of normal stature at rest or with minimal exercise, the lower airspaces are better ventilated than the apical airspaces. This is fortunate, since pulmonary artery flow is also gravity dependent and greater at the lung bases.

Microscopically, the alveoli are predominantly lined by very thin Type 1 epithelial cells with a few Type 2 cells which produce surfactant. In the interstitium there are elastic and collagen fibers and other cells, but most importantly from a gas exchange viewpoint, an abundance of pulmonary capillaries.[9] Each capillary is distensible but only large enough to allow normal red cells to travel through. In the alveolar wall, there is minimal distance and tissue between the capillary and the alveolar gas on either side of the capillary. Thus, the multiple capillaries in the alveolar wall exchange O_2 and CO_2 with the alveoli on both sides.

The large airways are lined with cilia, epithelial cells with underlying smooth muscles, fibrous tissue and cartilage. As airways become smaller, cartilage rings disappear and they become more collapsible and dependent on their surrounding pressures. With loss of alveolar tissue which tethers the airways and elastic recoil pressure, as in emphysema, the intrathoracic airway wall become more compressible during coughing or forceful exhalation. A few mucus-secreting goblet cells line the airways, but the majority of epithelial cells contain beating cilia, which through "clever" contortions, sweep inhaled and deposited debris and mucus from the terminal bronchioles to the trachea, where they are dumped into the gastrointestinal tract or coughed out. There are no cilia in the acini.

HEART AND PULMONARY CIRCULATION

For good reasons of economy and efficiency, the heart and lungs share the thorax and are intimately related. The volume of the heart and great vessels is relatively small in normal health but can double or triple in magnitude with heart disease. Thus, cardiomegaly, pulmonary edema and pleural effusions can markedly reduce the available space for the lung and cause restriction of the lung.

The pulmonary arteries are less muscular than systemic arteries. Soon after leaving the right ventricle, right and left main pulmonary arteries parallel the bronchi and bronchioles, branching with them all the way to the acini. There the arterioles profusely branch into the abundant airspace capillaries. Pulmonary venules and veins collect the pulmonary capillary blood and return the better oxygenated but lesser carbonated blood to the left atrium along routes separate from the pulmonary arteries and airways. A very small portion of pulmonary arteriolar blood can bypass the capillaries (i.e., shunt) and move directly to pulmonary veins and the left heart.

The filling of the airspace capillaries is variable and is dependent on several factors: including gravity and the state of activity of the subject. Normally, in the upright position at rest, most of the pulmonary capillaries are not filled with blood. Due to the low systolic and diastolic pressures in the pulmonary arteries, the apices are perfused much less than the lung bases. However, during exercise, they are increasingly filled with blood as cardiac output and pulmonary artery blood pressure rise. Disease states, such as pulmonary emboli, or the destruction of the capillary bed by emphysema, fibrosis or pulmonary vasculopathy can markedly reduce delivery of blood through the lung. This reduces the ability of the lung to transfer CO_2 from the blood to the airspaces and, especially, O_2 from the airspaces to the blood. In such states, it seems much more sensible and correct to term these deficiencies as "loss of pulmonary capillary vasculature" rather than as "loss of alveolar surface" as the "surface of most importance" is usually the quantity of red cells ready to load O_2 and unload CO_2 within the capillaries, not the epithelial surface of the alveoli. It should be added that the term "vascular" also includes anemia, carboxyhemoglobinemia or reduced cardiac output.

There are two other circulations to note. Lymphatics drain fluid from the acini of both lungs in unknown volumes and empty into the right or main lymphatic ducts and systemic veins. The thoracic aorta sends multiple branches to the thorax: intercostal arteries (which nourish the intercostal muscles), diaphragmatic arteries (which nourish the diaphragm) and bronchial arteries (which nourish the airways). The drainage of the bronchial arteries may pass eventually to either the right or the left sides of the heart.

MATCHING OR MISMATCHING OF VENTILATION AND PERFUSION

Matching of Ventilation and Perfusion in the Lung

For proper exchange of O_2 and CO_2 within the lung, ventilated gas must enter and exit perfused airspaces and blood must flow through the ventilated airspace capillaries from the right heart to the left heart. The following diagrams attempt to show such normal matching and a few examples of poor matching of ventilation to perfusion. From top to bottom in these diagrams, consider that the green airways extend from a point (mouth) and shaft (trachea and bronchi) of a giant thumb-tack or trumpet without valves through a small bell (bronchioles) to the airspaces, also in green, thinly covering a large thinly-painted magenta area (half the size of a tennis court) of pulmonary capillaries. The airways are primarily one-way streets, changing directions back and forth with each breath, while in the airspaces (alveoli, alveolar sacs, and alveolar ducts) diffusion predominates. Below, the right heart pumps purple blood containing O_2 lower-saturated hemoglobin (about 3/4 saturated at rest and ¼ saturated during intense exercise) through the pulmonary arteries and arterioles to the entire magenta area and the left heart receives red blood containing O_2 well-saturated blood from the pulmonary venules and veins. Across the entire "court", the thin layer of blood within the pulmonary capillaries becomes more bright red as it gives up a small fraction of its total CO_2 content to the airspace gas and receives, in exchange, nearly similar quantities of O_2. The systemic circulation is not shown.

It may be useful to consider at this time the importance of the matching of ventilation to lung perfusion. The theoretically worst matching, incompatible with life, would occur if the right lung were well-ventilated but not perfused and the left lung were well perfused but not ventilated. The right lung would have complete dead-space ventilation whereas the left lung would have complete shunting so that there would be no gas exchange. When lung contains air but is not adequately ventilated that is considered to be poor distribution of ventilation or maldistribution of ventilation. We can estimate maldistribution of ventilation non-invasively in the pulmonary laboratory. The quantification and distribution of lung perfusion requires other techniques. In real life, lung areas which are well ventilated but underperfused can be considered to have high wasted ventilation, poor ventilatory efficiency, or high ventilatory inefficiency, or high alveolar ventilation (V) to perfusion (Q). Such a person would have a high V/Q or high dead space ventilation. In contrast, lung areas which are well perfused but under ventilated can be considered have shunt-like effect or low V/Q. The term "shunt" should be reserved for situations inside or outside the lung where there is no gas exchange into the blood flowing into the left ventricle. The term "shunt-like" can be used for situations in which there is inadequate but not absent ventilation to pulmonary artery blood.

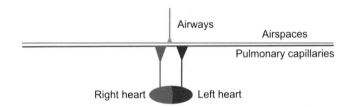

Figure 2-22 Normal lung with normal ventilation and perfusion. The airways are depicted as the shaft and point of a giant thumb-tack or trumpet without valves. The airspaces, also in green, normally cover an area half the size of a tennis court. The capillary surface area (magenta) is proportionally very large. The right and left heart are depicted below, the right heart pumping out violet blood (with 75% saturated oxyhemoglobin at rest, falling to below 25% with intense exercise) and the left heart receiving 95-98% saturated (red) blood regardless of level of exercise unless there are serious gas exchange problems. The systemic circulation is not shown. The airspace and capillary surfaces match well.

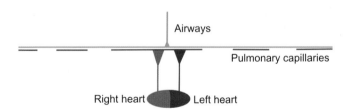

Figure 2-23 Lung with high V/Q areas. The alveoli are well ventilated but poorly perfused because the capillaries have been destroyed or obstructed. Considering the matching of the entire lung, the lung is over-ventilated so that extraction of O_2 from the atmosphere and return of CO_2 to the atmosphere is reduced. Thus, there is increased ventilation of dead space (unperfused lung) so that ventilation is not efficient. Mixed-expired CO_2 is likely to be low due to the reduced perfusion of well-ventilated airspaces. However, the red pulmonary venous and systemic arterial blood is well-saturated with O_2. Such a condition could occur with pulmonary emboli, or primary pulmonary hypertension associated with pulmonary vasculopathy. If measured, pulmonary artery pressure is likely to be increased.

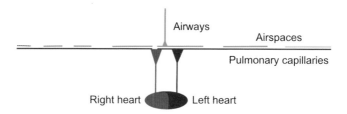

Figure 2-24 Lung with low V/Q areas. These lungs are poorly ventilated but well-perfused and are hence labeled as low V/Q. There is no increase of dead-space ventilation, but there is an increased perfusion of poorly ventilated lung. Consequently, the magenta-red blood returning to the left heart and the systemic circulation has low oxyhemoglobin saturation. Such areas can occur with atelectasis or pneumonia or malignancy or obesity or any other condition when the lung is not properly ventilated and perfusion persists to the under-ventilated areas of the lung. With obesity, the effect may be intermittent as a deep inspiration may relieve the atelectasis and hypoxemia.

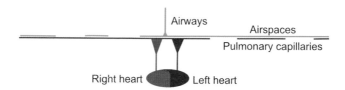

Figure 2-25 Lung with both high V/Q and low V/Q areas. Some portions of the lung are well ventilated and poorly perfused and other areas are poorly ventilated and well-perfused. This situation can occur in a variety of conditions, when perfusion fails to decrease in parallel with ventilation or ventilation fails to decrease in parallel with perfusion. There are both increased dead-space ventilation and hypoxemia. This can occur with either obstructive or restrictive lung disease or with left heart failure and may be partially reversible.

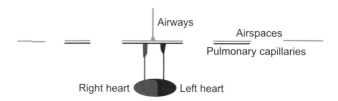

Figure 2-26 Lung with normal V/Q and high V/Q areas. This lung has lost structure, both airspaces and capillaries and is ventilating areas that are not perfused. There is no hypoxemia but dead space is increased and ventilation is inefficient. There may be more than one disease process in this patient.

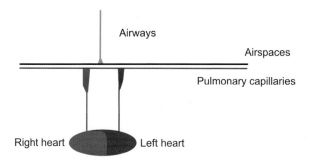

Figure 2-27 Restrictive lung disease. There are parallel losses of airspaces and capillaries. This could be due to lung resection, a large pleural effusion, malignancy or an immunologic disease.

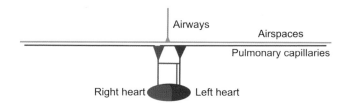

Figure 2-28 Extrapulmonary right to left shunt causing some abnormal desaturation of the systemic arterial blood. Ventilation is normal and adequate and not the cause of hypoxemia.

REFERENCES

1. Hansen JE. Unpublished observations.
2. Cotes JE. Lung function: Assessment and Application in Medicine, 4th edition. Oxfo rd: Blackwell; 1979.
3. Crapo RO, Morris AH, Clayton PD, et al. Lung volumes in healthy nonsmoking adults. *Bull Europ Physiopath Resp*. 1982;18:419-25.
4. Quanjer PhH, Tammeling GJ, Cotes JE, et al. Lung volumes and ventilatory flows. Report Working Party "Standardizatioin of Lung Function Tests", European Community for Steel and Coal and European Respiratory Society. *Eur Respir J*. 1993;6(Suppl16):5-40.
5. Gutierrez C, Ghezzo RH, Abboud RT, et al. Reference values of pulmonary function tests for Canadian Caucasians. *Can Respir J*. 2004;11:414-24.
6. Weibel ER. Morphometry of the Human Lung. New York: Springer; 1963. pp. 151.
7. Silverton RE. Gross fixation methods used in the study of pulmonary emphysema. *Thorax*, 1965;20:289-97. (Quote of Laennec)
8. Gough J, Wentworth JE. The use of thin sections of entire organs in morbid anatomical studies. *J Roy Micr Soc*. 1949;98:231-40.
9. Fishman AP. Pulmonary diseases and disorders. New York: McGraw-Hill; 1980.

10. Hansen JE, Ampaya EP, Bryant GH. Branching pattern of airways and airspaces of a single human terminal bronchiole. *J Appl Physiol*. 1975;38:983-9.

11. Hansen JE, Ampaya EP. Lung morphometry: a fallacy in the use of the counting principle. *J Appl Physiol*. 1974;37:951-4.

12. Hansen JE, Ampaya EP. Human airspace shapes, sizes, areas, and volumes. *J Appl Physiol*. 1975;38:990-5.

13. Paiva M, Lacquest LM, van der Linden LP. Gas transport in a model derived from the Hansen-Ampaya anatomical data of the human lung. *J Appl Physiol*. 1976;41:115-9.

14. Glazier JB, Hughes JM, Maloney JE, et al. Vertical gradient of alveolar size in lungs of dogs frozen intact. *J Appl Physiol*. 1967;23:694-705.

3 Preparation for Testing

INTRODUCTION

Lung function measurements can be made in clinics or wards by dedicated personnel or by individuals who have many other responsibilities. In surveys or the pulmonary function laboratory they are usually made by well-trained and dedicated personnel. Equipment may be portable or fixed in laboratories. This chapter primarily considers the use of fixed equipment and personnel dedicated to pulmonary function testing but the principles are reasonable wherever lung function is tested. Gas cylinders must be certified by national agencies and be safely secured; gas regulators, manifolds and valves properly installed; and disposable mouthpieces, nose-clips and filters disposable for single patient use or properly sterilized between patients. Further recommendations can be found in the publications of the European Respiratory Society and American Thoracic Society.[1,2]

EQUIPMENT FOR MEASURING SPIROMETRIC VOLUMES AND FLOW, LUNG VOLUMES AND TRANSFER OF CARBON MONOXIDE

In all cases, the laboratory should utilize equipment which meets American Thoracic Society (ATS)[1] and European Respiratory Society standards[2] and test gases which meet high standards. It is necessary to follow the exact quality control procedures outlined by the equipment manufacturer. The assistance of nearby distributors or individuals with knowledge and experience of the specific device can be helpful and time-saving. Equipment should be recalibrated before use at the timing and intervals recommended by the manufacturer.[3]

Spirometry

The volumes, capacities and flows (flow rate is a redundant term) of the vital capacity can be measured with spirometers of many differing types. Volume-measurement spirometers can be bell over water wet spirometers (which are still available), or dry rolling seal, wedge or bellows which can also translate volumes into flows. Flow-measurement spirometers can use pneumotachographs, heated wire sensors, ultrasonic flow-heads, rotating vanes or turbines with translation of flows to volumes by electronic integration. Using the internet allows one to consider a number of manufacturers and distributors. Lung volumes and flow rates are reported at body temperature (37º C) and 100% saturation with H_2O (47 mmHg), e.g., BTPS. As any given volume of exhaled air quickly cools to room temperature with decrease in PH_2O from 47 mmHg to the saturated pressure at ambient room temperature 22 mmHg at 22º C (e.g., ATPS), the volume of air exhaled is corrected by approximately 6-9%. The volume of gas in a spirometer must then be multiplied by that factor to correct the spirometer gas volumes and flows (ATPS) to the lung gas volumes and flows (BTPS). As noted previously the following can be calculated from measurements of VT, IRV and ERV. IC = VT + IRV; VC = IC + ERV. Also, not measured by spirometry alone, TLC = VC + RV, TLC = IC + FRC and FRC = RV + ERV.

Total Lung Capacity, Functional Residual Capacity, and Residual Volume

Measurement of total lung volumes is restful for the patient, but somewhat more complex than spirometry alone and requires an indirect measurement of the RV or TLC in the pulmonary laboratory.[4] Outside of the pulmonary function laboratory, the TLC can be directly calculated from PA and lateral chest radiographs taken in full inspiration. In the pulmonary laboratory, TLC is usually measured by adding together the FRC volume and IC volume. The IC is determined from spirometry; while the FRC is directly measured by plethysmography (body box), N_2 washout, or He dilution. The RV is calculated as the FRC minus the ERV. In all three methods, subject is "switched to" the measuring device near the FRC, with corrections added or subtracted for "switch in" errors when the "switch" in differs from normal quietend-expiration. Again, referral to the internet allows one to consider a number of manufacturers, distributors and costs of operation. With N_2 washout, 100% O_2 is required; with He dilution, gas cylinders with known quantities of He, N_2 and O_2 are required.

Diffusing Capacity of the Lung (DLCO), also Identified as Transfer Factor of CO for the Lung (TLCO)

Measurement of DLCO or TLCO and effective alveolar volume (VA') requires certified gas cylinders, special valves near the mouthpiece and the requirement to trap a portion of exhaled gas for CO and an inert tracing gas for measurement of pressures or quantities with a gas chromatograph or the ability to continuously record the pressures or concentrations of CO and the inert gas (usually methane) of the exhaled gas. The inhaled volume of a gas (with known concentrations of CO and the inert tracer), time of breath holding and exhaled volume must also be timed and known.

Publications from Salt Lake City experts using multiple volume, flow and DLCO measuring devices indicate the variability in accuracy and reproducibility which can be attributed to devices from several manufacturers and not due to personnel factors.[5,6]

PERSONNEL

It is highly recommended that personnel making pulmonary function measurements be well-trained and continue to make many measurements every week. It is difficult to maintain high quality standards and make useful and reliable measurements of lung function when either the equipment or the personnel making the measurements are infrequently used. A minimum of 4-6 subjects or patients should be measured every week; ideally that number or more should be measured every working day.

A recent publication describes the quality of tracings obtained in general practice settings in Switzerland which required spirometry training, high quality spirometers, and automated feedback and quality control. In the nearly 30,000 spirometries (usually ≤ 5 tracings each) collected and later analyzed by pulmonologists, 34% were graded as A, 7 % as B, 19% as C, 28% as D and 12% as F, indicating the challenges in obtaining quality spirometric tracings without dedicated personnel.[7]

REQUESTING THE TEST

If tests are not part of a survey, they should be specifically ordered by a well-qualified health professional. The request should state the primary diagnosis, any important secondary diagnoses and the reasons for testing. If the patient is taking short-acting bronchodilators, they should ordinarily be withheld for 6-8 hours. Ideally, the patients should stop smoking for 4 hours before testing. Other medications should be continued.

OBTAINING PATIENT OR SUBJECT HISTORY AND CONSENT

The subject being tested should fill out a questionnaire, with assistance if necessary.[8] If at all possible the questionnaire should be given in the language used by the subject/patient. The patient should record their gender and ethnicity or race, which is desirable in selecting normal reference values. The questionnaire should have space for the patient to state his/her primary symptom and its duration. Table 3-1 gives a suggested questionnaire.

The patient or subject should be told what measurements have been requested and are desirable to make. They should be advised that they have the right to question and/or refuse any measurement but that it is in their best interests to cooperate fully. They should be informed that, with their consent, their data without

Table 3-1	Questionnaire for Patient Coming to Pulmonary Laboratory or Evaluated During a Survey

Name, Last	Name, First	Medical or Survey ID #	Birth date: MM/DD/YY	Gender and race

Medical problem?

Questions	Answers	Comments
	YES ± NO	
Had lung test here before?		
Heart trouble or chest pain?		
Do you have shortness of breath? When?		
Do you cough?		
Do you raise sputum?		
Have you coughed blood?		
Do you have fever or sweats?		
Have you had TB?		
Recent weight loss?		
Do you wheeze or make noise with breathing?		
Have you had lung, heart or neck surgery? What? When?		
Are you exposed to dusts or fumes?		
Are you allergic? If so, comment		
Have you ever smoked tobacco? What kind?		
If yes, when started?		
If yes, when stopped?		
How many cigarettes, pipes, or cigars on average per day?		
Smoked today?		
List heart and lung meds		
When and what last lung med?		

any identification of them as individual, may be used for medical research purposes. The format and type of consent obtained will depend upon local circumstances and regulations.

ANTHROPOMETRIC MEASUREMENTS

Shoeless standing-tall height and weight without excess clothing or paraphernalia should be measured and recorded, preferably using the metric system. The patient's statement of their presumed weight and height should not be used. If there are significant deformities (kyphosis, scoliosis) or the patient is unable to stand upright the technician should so note and record the fingertip to fingertip distance and use that distance to replace standing height in predicting equations. If a hemoglobin measurement is available in the patient's records, the value should be recorded; if not a current measured hemoglobin value is desirable. It is also desirable to record a resting oximeter value from an earlobe, finger or forehead with annotation if the patient is breathing other than room air.

REFERENCES

1. American Thoracic Society. Standardization of spirometry, 1994 update. *Am J Respir Crit Care Med.* 1995;152:1107-36.
2. Miller MR, Hankinson J, Brusasco V, et al. Standardization of spirometry. *Eur Respir J.* 2005;26:319-38.
3. Clausen JL (Editor). Pulmonary Function Testing Guidelines and Controversies. New York: Academic Press; 1982;368.
4. Quanjer PH, Tammeling GJ, Cotes JE, et al. Lung volumes and forced ventilatory flows. Official statement of the European Respiratory Society. *Eur Respir J.* 1993;16(Suppl):5-40.
5. Jensen RL, Teeter JG, England RD, et al. Instrument accuracy and reproducibility in measurements of pulmonary function. *Chest.* 2007;132:388-95.
6. Jensen RL, Teeter JG, England RD, et al. Sources of long-term variability in measurements of lung function. *Chest.* 2007;132:396-402.
7. Leuppi JD, Miedinger D, Chhajed PN, et al. Quality of spirometry in primary care for case finding of airway obstruction in smokers. *Respiration.* 2010;79(6):469-74.
8. Yawn BP, Mapel DW, Mannino DM, et al. Development of the lung function questionnaire (LFQ) to identify airflow obstruction. *International Journal of COPD.* 2010;5:1-10.

4 Basic Spirometry

WHAT SPIROMETRY DOES AND DOES NOT MEASURE

A spirometer is the most basic and commonly used device for measuring lung function, whether for population surveys in the field, for clinical assessment of individual patients in the clinical pulmonary laboratory or hospital wards, or for evaluating normal subjects or patients in research laboratories. Spirometry is excellent for measuring airway obstruction, both expiratory and inspiratory, and for measuring changes over time or in response to interventions or therapy. It measures VC, but not RV, FRC or TLC, so although it can suggest, or even strongly suggest, restriction, it cannot alone identify or quantitate restriction. Once a restrictive process is proven by adequate reduction of TLC, spirometric measures can usually be used to follow the progression or regression of restriction. Spirometry cannot assess the presence or absence nor progression or regression of pulmonary vascular disease. However, since VC decreases with pulmonary edema or pleural effusions, laboratory or bedside spirometry can be useful in quickly assessing the regression or progression of left heart failure.

EQUIPMENT CALIBRATION

Each spirometer, whether measuring volume directly and flow indirectly (rolling seal, wedge, bell or other) or measuring flow directly (pneumotachograph, heated wire, turbine or other) should be certified to meet ATS standards.[1,2] Volume spirometers should be checked for leaks weekly and flow spirometers should be calibrated at least daily, using a 3.00 L or other size syringe of known volume. The room temperature and barometric pressure should be known; either directly measured, or obtained from a local airport or government agency. Calibration should follow manufacturer's directions, but usually consists of six or more complete inhalations or exhalations into the spirometer using complete and smooth cycles. Each cycle must be very slow, very fast or of intermediate velocities. The usual acceptable range for repeated measurements at all three velocities is ±3%.

DISPLAYING TIME VERSUS VOLUME AND VOLUME VERSUS FLOW

Time versus Volume Display

Most spirometers display time on the X axis, usually moving from left to right. Volume is displayed on the Y axis, with TLC either superiorly or inferiorly and RV necessarily the opposite. Slow or unforced vital capacities can be measured initially or later. For all measurements, the patient should be seated comfortably upright on a chair so he/she can bend forward as necessary. A nose clamp is applied and the patient asked to sniff. If air cannot pass through the nose, the clamp position is satisfactory. A clean mouthpiece of comfortable size, often with a flange between the lips and the teeth is placed in the mouth and the patient instructed to hold the mouthpiece tightly so that no air can leak around it. A low resistance filter may also be placed in line to reduce the likelihood of contamination.

Unforced VC

As the patient breathes comfortably, resting tidal volumes are recorded. The patient is then asked to take a maximal inhalation, hold it momentarily, and then asked to exhale completely but not necessarily rapidly until he/she cannot exhale further (Figure 4-1). The expiratory maneuver should last several seconds in normal adults, and longer in those with significant airway obstruction. This maneuver can be followed with a deep or partial inhalation (Figure 4-2).

Adding Volume Versus Flow Display

Most spirometers can also display concurrently volume on the X-axis and flow, both expiratory and inspiratory on the Y-axis. Time signals may or may not be evident.

Forced VC

The patient is asked to return to resting tidal breathing, then inhale maximally, pause very briefly, and then exhale with maximal effort for at least six seconds. If there is no further change in expired volume after 6 seconds, a full forced inspiration follows. If expiratory flow continues after 6 seconds, it is ordinarily continued until the flow ceases and the volume plateaus, or for 10-15 seconds. It is usually unnecessary or unwise to continue forced exhalation longer than that, because forced exhalation impedes the flow of blood back to the thorax and may result in light-headedness due to impaired blood flow to the brain. The forced maneuver should be repeated at least two more times to obtain adequate duplicate measures, but rarely repeated more than six times to avoid patient frustration and exhaustion. Such forced maneuvers are displayed in figures 4-3 and 4-4. At least once, after measuring the slow or forced

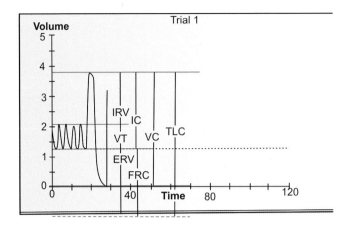

Figure 4-1 Spirometric volume versus time display, from left to right, of tidal breathing, a maximal inspiration, a slow maximal expiration and a partial inspiration in a normal subject. Horizontal red lines separate volumes and capacities. RV, FRC and TLC cannot be measured from spirometry alone. (ERV = expiratory reserve volume, FRC = functional residual capacity, IC = inspiratory capacity, IRV = inspiratory reserve volume, RV = residual volume, TLC = total lung capacity, VC = vital capacity, VT = tidal volume.)

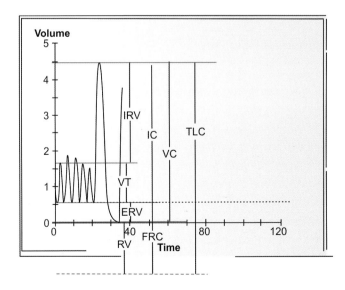

Figure 4-2 Spirometric volume versus time display, from left to right in a more obese otherwise normal subject. Note smaller ERV and higher IC/ERV ratio abbreviations as in (Figure 4-1).

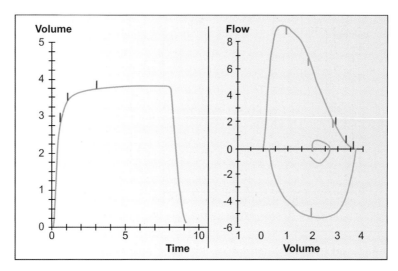

Figure 4-3 Forced expiratory and forced inspiratory maneuvers on time-volume (left) and volume-flow (right) tracings of a 37-year-old man. On the volume-flow tracing, resting tidal breathing with IRV, VT and ERV are not marked but can also be identified. On both tracings, upward tick marks colored red can be seen at 0.5 sec, 1.0 sec and 3.0 sec. On the volume-flow tracing, inward green tick marks during forced expiration indicate the $FEF_{25\%}$, $FEF_{50\%}$ and $FEF_{75\%}$ while the green tick mark on forced inspiration indicates the $FIF_{50\%}$. Some other values are: $FEV_{0.5}$ = 2.95 L, FEV_1 = 3.30 L, FEV_3 = 3.62 L, FEV_6 = 3.63 L, FVC = 3.70 L, peak flow = 9.2 L/sec, IRV = 1.90 L, VT = 0.80 L, ERV = 1.00 L. [Abbreviations as in Figure 4-1 plus FEF = forced expiratory flows at several percentages of the forced vital capacity (FVC), FEV_x = forced expiratory volumes at several times.]

vital capacity, a forceful rapid measurement should be made of the inspiratory vital capacity and flow from RV to TLC. Ideally, the best inspiratory vital capacity should approximately be the best expiratory vital capacity. If the inspiratory VC and FVC measures differ by more than 5%, it means that the patient did not exhale or inhale completely with the smaller VC maneuver.

In adults without moderate or more severe obstruction, the best slow vital capacity and best forced vital capacity should also differ by less than five percent. With more severe obstruction, the slow vital capacity may exceed the forced vital capacity due to compression of the intrathoracic airways by the high intrathoracic pressures generated during the forced maneuvers.

On the volume-time or flow-volume recordings (Figures 4-1 to 4-4), the VT, ERV, IRV, IC and VC can be easily and directly measured. It is important to note that for VC the maximal value from any maneuver is taken as valid and reported. On the

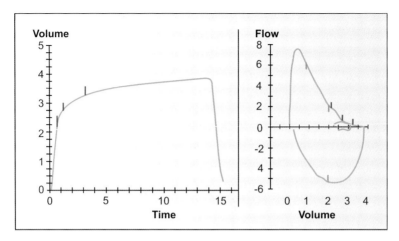

Figure 4-4 Forced expiratory and forced inspiratory maneuvers on time-volume (left) and volume-flow (right) tracings of an 83-year-old man. On the volume-flow tracing, resting tidal breathing with IRV, VT and ERV are not marked but can also be identified. On both tracings, upward tick marks colored red can be seen at 0.5 sec, 1.0 sec and 3.0 sec. On the volume-flow tracing, inward green tick marks during forced expiration indicate the $FEF_{25\%}$, $FEF_{50\%}$ and $FEF_{75\%}$ while the green tick mark on forced inspiration indicates the $FIF_{50\%}$. Some other values are: FEV_1 = 2.72 L, FEV_3 = 3.27 L, FEV_6 = 3.53 L, FVC = 3.82 L, peak flow = 7.6 L/sec, IRV = 2.32 L, VT = 0.70 L, ERV = 0.80 L.

other hand the measures of VT, ERV, IRV and IC are the average of values rather than the individually highest averages so that the values of IC and ERV should add up to the same value as the VC.

On the volume-time display, the $FEV_{0.5}$, FEV_1, FEV_3, FEV_6, FVC and any other timed volume can be easily and accurately measured (Figures 4-1 and 4-2). Although not commonly done, flows can be accurately measured at any time on the time-volume display as the slope of the recorded curve at any one time. Such a line can be drawn parallel to a short segment of the curve, or as a straight line between two points on the curve. For example, the slope at 50% of the FVC is the $FEF_{50\%}$. The line exactly connecting the points at 25% of the FVC and at 75% of the FVC measures the $FEF_{25-75\%}$ flow for that maneuver. If a recorded line on the time-volume display is exactly linear, it means that flow is constant over that time period. If the line is linear and parallel to the X-axis, that constant flow is "zero". Note the difference in tracings with aging.

Maximum Voluntary Ventilation

The direct maximum voluntary ventilation (MVV) (previously known as the maximal breathing capacity) is measured by having the patient breathe in and out as forcefully as possible for 12-15 seconds (Figure 4-5). The spirometer tracing shows the tidal volumes and breathing frequency while a mechanical or electronic device sums the total inspiratory OR expiratory volumes over the same 12-second period. There is often a tendency for technicians to have the patient breath too rapidly and too shallowly. If the subject breathes at a frequency above 60-80 breaths per minute during the maneuver, it is suggested that the technicians tutor the patients to breathe more deeply and at a slower frequency. Fortunately, however, as shown by figure 4-6 in a cooperative patient, the MVV is only minimally affected by breathing frequency.

The measurement of the direct MVV over a 12-second period is useful to assess not only the lungs but also the patient's strength, coordination and ability to cooperate (Figures 4-5 and 4-6). As such, it may be useful in assessing preoperatively a borderline patient's operability or prior to exercise testing to help ascertain whether or not a patient is ventilatory limited during exercise.[3] The indirect MVV can be calculated by multiplying the FEV_1 by a factor. Although the factor of 35 times the FEV_1 was initially recommended for calculation of the MVV,[4] the authors only reported that the $FEV_1 \times 35$ was highly correlated with the direct MVV. However, any numeric factor used would also have been highly correlated. In our and others' experience, 40 is a better factor to multiply times FEV_1 in L to calculate indirect MVV in L/min for normal individuals and patients with obstructive lung disease.[5,6] With interstitial lung disease, the indirect MVV so calculated often greatly exceeds the direct MVV due to a high elastic recoil of the lungs, strong breathing muscles and

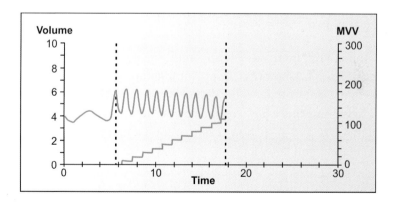

Figure 4-5 Direct maximum voluntary ventilation (MVV) measured for 12 seconds in an 83-year-old man. After ~5.5 seconds of quiet breathing maximal inspiratory and expiratory efforts are made at a frequency of 60 cycles per minute. The upper tracing show the actual volumes in L on the left Y-axis while the concurrent lower tracing shows the inspiratory volumes divided by 30 on the right Y-axis to express the value in L/min.

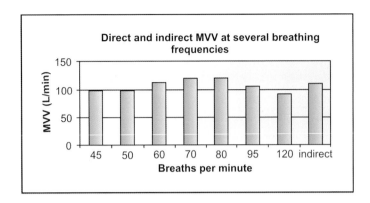

Figure 4-6 Maximum voluntary ventilation measured at 7 breathing frequencies. There is some dependence of MVV on breathing frequency, with frequencies of 60 to 80 per minute giving the highest values. The indirect MVV, calculated by FEV_1 of 2.72 L times 40 equals 109 L/min; quite similar to the average volumes/min of the direct MVV.

high breathing frequency.[3] With severe obesity, the direct MVV is often lower than $40 \times FEV_1$ due to the inertia of rapidly changing the direction of movement of the thorax and abdomen.

Before examining patterns of volume and flow further, it is reasonable to consider the variability of these variables in apparently normal populations.

VARIABILITY OF DATA IN INDIVIDUALS THOUGHT TO BE NORMAL

Figure 4-7 shows FEV_1 from over 700 apparently healthy never-smoking black men sorted by age. Figure 4-8 shows FVC from over 1,300 apparently healthy Latin women sorted by height. Figure 4-9 shows the deviations of actual FEV_1 from predicted FEV_1 for healthy never-smoking white women after accounting for differences in age and height. Figures 4-10 and 4-11 show scatter around a narrow age and height range for several volumes and flows for 45-47-year-old never-smoking white men 177.5–180 cm tall. Figure 4-12 shows variability of $FEF_{25-75\%}$ in 20 never-smoking black women within 1.0 cm of height all of the 3rd decade of age, when differences between subjects in lung volumes and flow rates are minimized.

From these figures it is apparent that there is marked variability in apparently normal never-smoking adults within narrow age ranges and narrow height ranges in FEV_1 and FVC (Figures 4-7 and 4-8). Even with excellent predicting equations accounting for age and height, considerable variability remains for FEV_1 (Figure 4-9). As one can see, the range of actual values for FEV_1 (or FEV_3, FEV_6, or FVC) on the

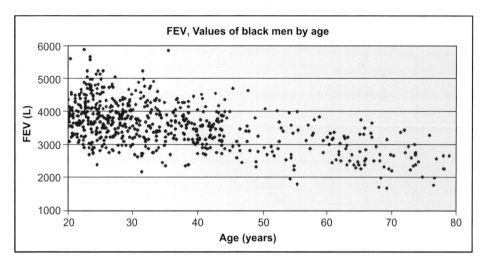

Figure 4-7 FEV$_1$ measurements of 700 NHANES-3 never-smoking normal black men of varying heights arranged by age. Note wide scatter of values.

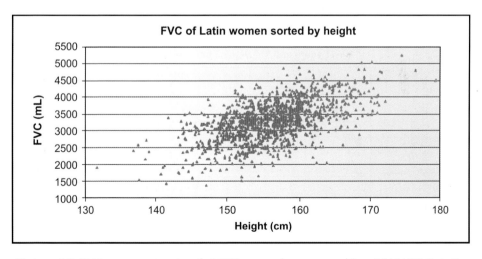

Figure 4-8 FVC measurements of 1,300 normal never-smoking NHANES-3 Latin women aged 20-78 years, arranged by heights. Note wide scatter of values.

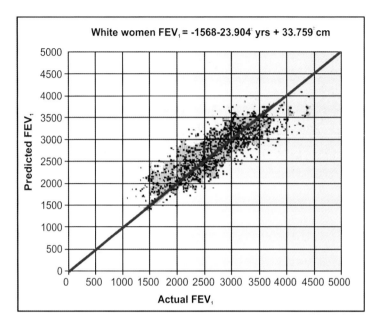

Figure 4-9 FEV$_1$ measurements of 1,400 never-smoking NHANES-3 white women compared with the predicted values of the same population. The equation FEV$_1$ (mL) = −1548 − 23.904 × age in years + 33.759 x height in cm minimizes deviations of actual from predicted values for both X- and Y-axes.

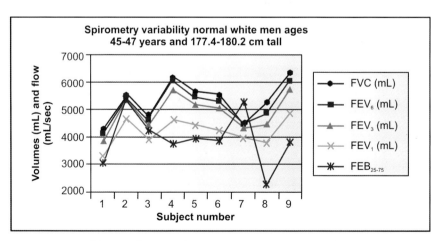

Figure 4-10 Timed-lung-volume and FEF$_{25-75\%}$ measurements of the 9 normal never-smoking NHANES-3 white men of similar age (45-47 years) and height (177.4-180.2 cm). Note the moderate variability of the lung volumes and the higher variability of the FEF$_{25-75\%}$ measurements.

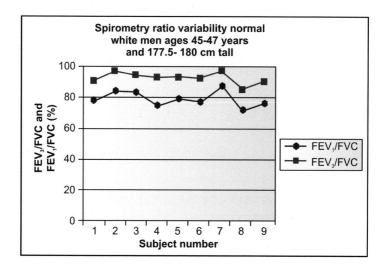

Figure 4-11 %FEV$_1$/FVC and %FEV$_3$/FVC ratio values from the same men as in Figure 4-10. Note the much lesser variability of these ratios than the absolute values from which they are derived.

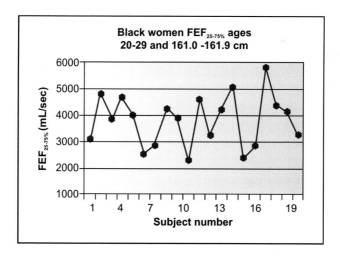

Figure 4-12 FEF$_{25-75\%}$ in 20 consecutive never-smoking NHANES-3 black women of ages 20-29 and heights of 161.0-161.9 cm. In this age range, FVC and FEV$_1$ values are relatively stable while variability of FEF$_{25-75\%}$ is considerably higher.

X-axis can exceed 1500 mL for a given predicted volume of FEV_1, FEV_3, FEV_6 or FVC on the Y-axis. When the range of ages and heights (Figures 4-10 to 4-12) in individuals of the same gender and ethnicity are markedly limited, the variability of volumes is moderate (FVC, FEV_1, FEV_3 and FEV_6), the ratio of volumes to volumes is much less (FEV_1/FVC and FEV_3/FVC) but the variability of the $FEF_{25-75\%}$ (a flow/volume) is very high. This pattern of variability is inherent in all published predicting equations and suggests some caution in identifying and quantifying obstruction and even more caution when we use volume to diagnose and quantify restriction. But there is hope. In table 4-1 and the following figures the most useful flow and volume measurements will be emphasized.

SPIROMETRIC MEASUREMENTS WORTH RECORDING, VIEWING AND INTERPRETING

The patterns of airflow obstruction seen on volume-flow axes are also easy to recognize. Normally, in early youth, the forced expiratory tracing may bow outward; soon thereafter, the flow declines in a relatively straight line from peak flow early in the forced maneuvers to zero flow at the end of the maneuver (Figures 4-13 and 4-14). With normal aging flow tends to sag downward or become concave (Figures 4-3 and 4-4). With increasing obstruction at any age (Figures 4-15 to 4-17) the forced expiratory flow patterns become markedly depressed so that forced expiratoy flow is less than expiratory flow during quiet breathing in the tidal volume range.

Table 4-1 Spirometric Measurements Likely to be of Clinical Value
Slow vital capacity (SVC)
Forced vital capacity (FVC) and/or Forced expiratory volume in 6 seconds (FEV_6)
Inspiratory capacity (IC)
Expiratory reserve volume (ERV)
Forced expiratory volume in 1 second (FEV_1)
Forced expiratory volume in 3 seconds (FEV_3)
%FEV_1/FVC or %FEV_1/FEV_6
%FEV_3/FVC or %FEV_3/FEV_6 or 1-FEV_3/FVC or 1-FEV_3/FEV_6
Peak expiratory flow or mid-expiratory flow
Peak inspiratory flow
Maximum voluntary ventilation (MVV), direct

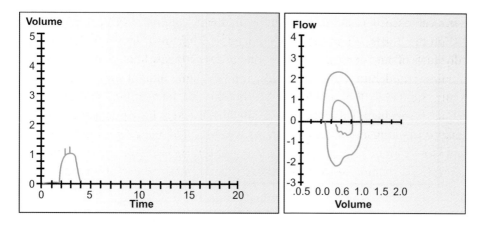

Figure 4-13 Time versus volume and volume versus flow tracings of a normal 9-year-old boy, 117 cm tall and weighing 32 kg. Expiratory flow is mildly concave in volume versus flow tracing.

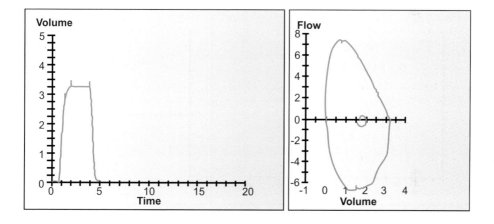

Figure 4-14 Time versus volume and volume versus flow tracings of a normal 18-year-old adolescent male. Decline in expiratory flow is quite linear in volume versus flow tracing.

Volumes

In patients, it is reasonable to obtain the best slow or unforced VC and necessary to obtain the best FVC, since the SVC may be larger than the FVC when there is significant airway obstruction. If there is no airway obstruction and the SVC differs from the FVC by more than a few percent, the spirometry is of low quality. This may be due to circumstances beyond the control of the patient or technician. The

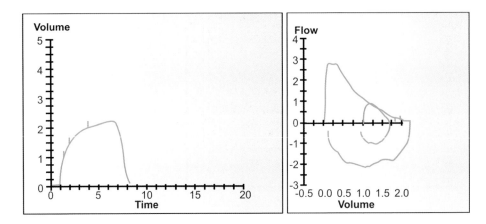

Figure 4-15 Time versus volume and volume versus flow tracings of a 70-year-old woman, 160 cm tall and weighing 99 kg. $FEV_1/FVC = 65\%$. Mild airway obstruction with low respiratory reserve volume.

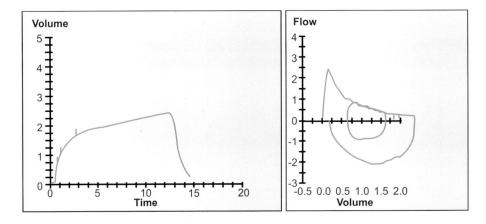

Figure 4-16 Time versus volume and volume versus flow tracings of an 80-year-old woman, 147 cm tall and weighing 55 kg. FVC is normal. $FEV_1/FVC = 46\%$. Moderately severe airway obstruction.

FEV_1, FEV_3 and FEV_6 are usually readily available. In normal to mild airway disease the FVC is probably preferable to the FEV_6, but the latter is less stressful and more reproducible for many patients with moderate to severe airway obstruction. The FVC maneuvers longer than 12-15 seconds run the risk of inducing lightheadedness or fainting due to reduced cerebral blood flow (because high intrathoracic pressures impede the return of blood to the heart).

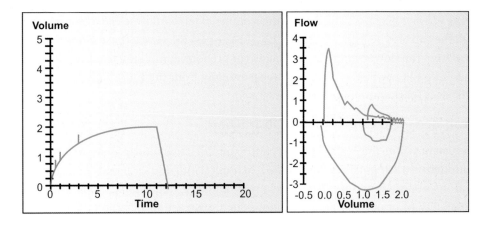

Figure 4-17 Time versus volume and volume versus flow tracings of a 73-year-old man, 175 cm tall and weighing 72 kg. FVC is 52% of predicted. $FEV_1/FVC = 47\%$. Severe airway obstruction.

Expiratory Reserve Volume and Inspiratory Capacity

These important measures (ERV and IC) are readily available from the time-volume displays and/or flow volume displays, but, unfortunately, are often not tabulated or interpreted. Each is best averaged from several tracings so that their sum equals the best VC or FVC. Nowadays, reduction of VC and TLC are often due to obesity rather than intrinsic lung disease. A reduction in ERV is closely related to abdominal and thoracic obesity. In mildly overweight to moderately obese individuals, the IC normally increases as the ERV (and FRC) decreases.[7] In very extreme obesity, the IC may also be reduced. It is very useful to consider the actual IC. If the actual IC is 2/3 or more of the predicted VC, a reduction in VC (i.e., a low ERV) can usually be attributed to obesity rather than intrinsic lung disease. If it is less than 2/3 of the predicted VC, the likelihood of other causes of restriction increases.

Ratios of Timed Volumes

Laboratories tend to report the FEV_1/VC, defining VC as the largest of any measure of VC, whether forced or slow, expiratory or inspiratory. When there are significant differences between the FVC, SVC and IVC measures of vital capacity, the interpreter may calculate each one and consider how they may help define the patient's disorder(s). The FEV_1/FEV_6 can usually be substituted for the FEV_1/FVC; with severe obstruction, they will differ. The FEV_3 is useful for comparison to the FEV_6 or FVC, since the $FVC-FEV_3$ or FEV_6-FEV_3 is the volume of airflow from the slower emptying airspaces and airways and thus these values are the optimal ones to assess small airways disease.[8] The ratio of this volume of late airflow to the total expiratory volume can also be expressed as $1\text{-}FEV_3/FEV_6$ or $1\text{-}FEV_3/FVC$. These ratios measure flow from the slower-emptying airspaces (or predominantly smaller airways) just as the FEV_1/FVC or FEV_1/FEV_6 ratios measure flow from the more rapidly emptying airspaces (or predominantly larger airways).

Peak Flows and Upper Airway Obstruction

It is useful to note the peak inspiratory and expiratory flows and to look carefully at the spirometric tracings if they are reduced. In normal individuals at mid-VC, expiratory and inspiratory flows are usually relatively equal. If not, one has to consider the possibility of upper airway obstruction. Such obstruction may be relatively fixed (e.g., tracheostomy strictures or damage, some neoplasms, laryngeal stenosis) or may be variable (e.g., evident only on forced exhalation or forced inhalation). If the obstruction is intrathoracic, it is likely to be most evident on forced exhalation since intrathoracic airways are compressed by high intrathoracic pressures secondary to the forced maneuver. If the obstruction is extrathoracic it is likely to be more evident on forced inhalation, since atmospheric pressure surrounding the neck exceeds airway pressure and tends to compress those airways outside the thorax. Since physicians and technicians tend to emphasize expiratory flow rather than inspiratory flow, it is important to train technicians so that when they encounter a patient with low peak inspiratory flow, they temporarily deemphasize expiratory flow and obtain at least one inspiratory tracing with maximal inspiratory effort. Good inspiratory flow on a single tracing strongly suggests that prior recorded low inspiratory flows were due to reduced inspiratory effort or weakness rather than upper airway obstruction.

With fixed upper airway obstruction both the expiratory flow and inspiratory flow tend to be near parallel for the early and mid-portions of the maneuvers (Figure 4-18). If a physician wishes to test the pattern of fixed upper airway obstruction, he/she need only breathe forcefully out for several seconds (from TLC to RV) and forcefully in for several seconds (from RV to TLC) through an endotracheal tube connected to a spirometer. It is next to impossible to increase inspiratory or expiratory flow to normal peak values when the large airway diameter is limited by such a tube or by upper airway narrowing. Note that when the endotracheal tube is no longer limiting flow in a maneuver, both expiratory and inspiratory flows move toward the no flow zero Y-axis.

Upper airway obstruction may be fixed or variable. Classically, fixed obstruction causes low flow during both inspiration and expiration (Figure 4-18). This flow is quite reproducible on repeated tracings since the flow cannot be increased by increasing the force of inspiration or expiration. Figure 4-19 illustrates a variable extrathoracic obstruction. Flow is markedly decreased during inspiration because

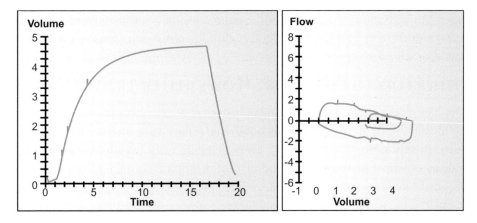

Figure 4-18 Time versus volume and volume versus flow tracings of a patient with a fixed upper airway obstruction. Note both slow rise and fall in time-volume tracing and nearly flat tracings in volume-flow tracings.

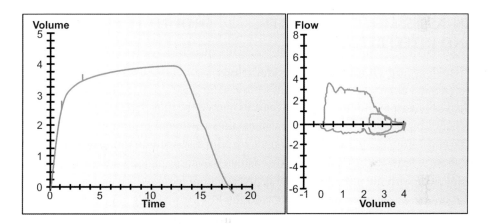

Figure 4-19 Time versus volume and volume versus flow tracings of a patient with a variable extrathoracic airway obstruction. Note the very low inspiratory flow in both tracings plus the moderate reduction of expiratory flow.

atmospheric pressure around the narrowed extrathoracic larynx or trachea is greater than pressure inside the constricted lumen. During expiration, intraluminal pressure is much higher than atmospheric pressure so that the lumen increases and early flow is only partially impeded. During late expiratory flow, compression of the intrathoracic airways limits flow, as occurs in normal adults. Classically, a variable intrathoracic obstruction causes a relatively flat plateau in early and mid-exhalation when the high intrathoracic pressure compresses the obstructed lumen, but little or no reduction in flow on inhalation because the obstruction tends to open when intrathoracic pressure is below atmospheric and intraluminal pressure.

OTHER FORCED EXPIRATORY FLOWS (FEF) OF LIMITED VALUES

The measures in table 4-2 are mostly of historical importance. There is minimal or no further information disclosed by obtaining, reporting or interpreting the values listed in this table. The $FEF_{200-1200}$ measurements were introduced and used as indices of effectiveness of coughing or raising sputum. In patients with severely reduced FVC, they often include flow far later in exhalation. Thus, the $FEF_{100-600}$ measurement was introduced. Overall, these measurements are less discriminating than peak expiratory flow measures.

Each of the FEF values is inherently a flow (e.g., L/sec or L/min) divided by a volume and thus has higher inherent variability in a population than does the FEV_1/FEV_6, FEV_1/FVC, FEV_3/FEV_6 or FEV_3/FVC. The next and later sections will further demonstrate the high inherent variability of the $FEF_{25-75\%}$ in normal populations.

AN ASSESSMENT OF THE $FEF_{25-75\%}$. SHOULD IT BE RECORDED AND INTERPRETED?

Historical and Theoretical Considerations

The $FEF_{25-75\%}$ was initially identified as and named the maximal mid-expiratory flow (MMEF) by Leuallan and Fowler.[9] It measures the mean expiratory flow between 25% and 75% of the forced vital capacity, i.e., the mid-volume (not mid-time) of the expiratory flow. In the desire to find sensitive measures of early airflow obstruction associated with air pollution, several investigators assessed several measures. At that time it was evident that the FVC and the FEV_1 were likely to be below the one-tailed 95% confidence limits in younger individuals, if they were less than 80% of mean predicted levels. Ignoring the variability of different spirometric measures,

Table 4-2	Spirometric Measurements Not Likely to be of Clinical Value
Forced expiratory flow from 100 to 600 mL ($FEF_{100-600}$)	
Forced expiratory flow from 200 to 1200 mL ($FEF_{200-1200}$)	
Forced expiratory flow at 25% of the VC ($FEF_{25\%}$)	
Forced expiratory flow at 50% of the VC ($FEF_{50\%}$)	
Forced expiratory flow at 75% of the VC ($FEF_{75\%}$)	
Forced expiratory flow at 25-75% of the VC ($FEF_{25-75\%}$)	
Forced expiratory flow at 75-85% of the VC ($FEF_{75-85\%}$)	

especially the very high variability of the $FEF_{25-75\%}$, some investigators promulgated the idea that a $FEF_{25-75\%}$ value below 80% of mean predicted was abnormal.[10,11] Against all logic and reality, this idea was widely accepted by many in the pulmonary and general medical community. It became commonplace for many physicians to interpret subjects with FEV_1, FVC and FEV_1/FVC within normal limits (e.g., above an arbitrary 80% of predicted) and with an $FEF_{25-75\%}$ below 80% as abnormal and indicative (or highly suggestive) of small airways disease. Later, many investigators and committees of major professional societies realized that considering 80% was not an inherent "cut-off" level, and that to consider any $FEF_{25-75\%}$ below 80% of predicted as abnormal was erroneous.[12-15] Despite this, physicians entering pulmonary training often interpret $FEF_{25-75\%}$ below 80% of mean predicted as indicative of small airways disease. It is time to examine the facts again.

First, the $FEF_{25-75\%}$ is a flow divided by a volume. Timed volumes have moderate population variability, while timed volumes divided by volumes have much less variability. Flows divided by volumes have inherent population variability. This is especially true since volumes like the FVC have quite high variability in a population of normal individuals of the same size, gender, age and ethnicity. Therefore, variability of any segment of a population is high so that the lower 95% confidence limits of $FEF_{25\%}$, $FEF_{50\%}$, $FEF_{75\%}$ and $FEF_{25-75\%}$ are invariably lower than 80% of mean predicted, especially in older individuals. Figure 4-10 showed the very high variability in 10 never-smoking white men all close to the same age, ethnicity, gender, and height. Figure 4-12 showed the very high variability of $FEF_{25-75\%}$ in 20 never-smoking black women of the same height and all in the 3rd decade of life, when FVC and FEV_1 values are most stable. Figure 4-20 shows differences in variability (measured as 95% confidence limits for lower limits of normal) in hundreds of normal never-smoking adult white women.[12] Specifically, for $FEF_{25-75\%}$, the highest LLN is 64% of mean predicted at age 20 and declines to ~42% at age 60, ~35% at age 70 and ~12% at age 80 years.

Second, it is reasonable to consider that the early part of the forced expiratory maneuver is predominantly limited by the larger airways, including the mouth, pharynx, larynx, trachea and major bronchi. Attempting to exhale forcefully through a small aperture confirms how this limits peak flow, $FEV_{0.5}$ and FEV_1. On the other hand, the end of the forced expiratory maneuver is predominantly limited by the late emptying airspaces and smaller airways. The low and very prolonged flow found in severe emphysema patients confirms this. The "middle" 50% usually includes both earlier and later parts of the forced expiratory maneuver.

Third, the $FEF_{25-75\%}$ does not usually evaluate "smaller airways" because it measures variable portions of the expiratory maneuver inherently dependent on the degree of airway obstruction as shown in figure 4-21. In normal adults, the $FEF_{25-75\%}$

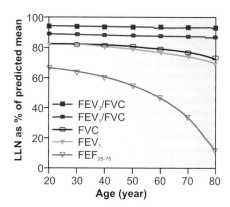

Figure 4-20 Lower limit of normal (95% confidence limits) derived from over 1,400 NHANES-3 never-smoking white women for these 5 spirometric measurements: FEV₃/FVC, FEV₁/FVC, FVC, FEV₁ and FEF$_{25-75\%}$. Note that the ratios of volumes have the least variability, absolute volumes have intermediate variability, and flows/volumes have the highest variability. Note FEF$_{25-75\%}$ LLN is never above 70% of mean predicted and declines rapidly with increasing age. The use of 80% of predicted to separate reduced flow (airway obstruction) from normal for all ages and measures is clearly not warranted.

measurement is finished before or very shortly after the FEV₁ measurement is finished (Figure 4-21, black tracing). Clearly in these cases, the FEF$_{25-75\%}$ measurement (with high inherent variability) adds nothing to the FEV₁/FVC measurement (with low inherent variability) but confusion. In patients with severe obstruction when the FEV₁/FVC is already markedly abnormal, the FEF$_{25-75\%}$ measures flow during the FEV₁ and well thereafter (Figure 4-21, red tracing). Thus the FEF$_{25-75\%}$ measurement is unnecessary. In cases with mild to moderate airway obstruction, both the FEV₁/FVC and the FEF$_{25-75\%}$ are below 95% confidence limits, so that the latter is again unnecessary (Figure 4-21, purple and blue tracings).

Fourth, there is a much better spirometric measurement available to assess smaller airways function. Logically that measure should occur during the latter half of the forced expiratory maneuver regardless of the degree of airway obstruction. The 1-FEV₃/FVC meets that criterion fairly well.[12] It is derived easily from measurement of the FEV₃ and FVC. The FVC-FEV₃ is the entire volume exhaled after 3 seconds, so that FVC-FEV₃/FVC or 1-FEV₃/FVC is ratio of the late expired volume divided by the entire expired volume.[12]

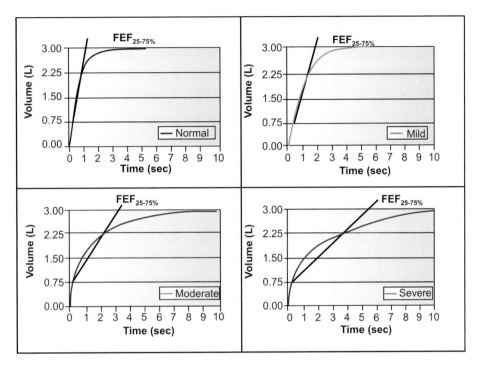

Figure 4-21 The FEF$_{25-75\%}$ measurements in four individuals of different ages and heights, each with an FVC of 3.00 L. The FVC volume has been divided into four quarters at 0.75, 1.50, 2.25 and 3.00 L. The diagonal tangents of the flow intersect the 25% and 75% volumes (i.e., the FEF$_{25-75\%}$ measurements) at differing times so that they reflect, early, mid or later flow in the forced expiration, depending on the degree of severity of the airflow obstruction.

Evidence and Analysis of Data

Not long ago we analyzed high-quality spirometric data collected by other investigators from a large number of never-smoking and current smoking adults in the NHANES-3.[12] We used the established equations of Hankinson et al.,[8] derived from several thousand NHANES-3 never-smoking population for mean and lower limit of normal (95% confidence limits) for FVC, FEV$_1$, FEV$_1$/FVC and FEF$_{25-75\%}$ for each ethnicity. For this same population we derived new reference equations for mean and lower limit of normal FEV$_3$/FVC values (95% confidence limits) from over 5,000 NHANES-3 never-smokers to evaluate 3,500 NHANES-3 current smoking adults. The most important data are presented in table 4-3. In line 1, note that of the 2,403 never-smoking subjects with normal FVC, FEV$_1$, FEV$_1$/FVC and FEV$_3$/FVC; only 1% had an abnormal FEF$_{25-75\%}$. This indicates that when the FVC, FEV$_1$, FEV$_1$/

FVC and FEV_3/FVC are normal, the $FEF_{25-75\%}$ is rarely below the LLN, and thus rarely of added use in detecting a statistically significant abnormality.

Probable False Positives

In line 2, although the FEV_1/FVC and FEV_3/FVC were normal, either the FVC or the FEV_1 was below the LLN, suggesting restrictive disease without obstruction. In 20% of these cases the $FEF_{25-75\%}$ was abnormal, despite the absence of statistically significant obstruction. Thus, in lung restriction, the $FEF_{25-75\%}$ may become abnormal despite the absence of significant airway obstruction.

Probable False Negatives

In line 3, obstruction was clearly present (both ratios of FEV_1/FVC and FEV_3/FVC reduced) and restriction absent (FVC and FEV_1 normal), yet in 42% the $FEF_{25-75\%}$ was normal, i.e., above the LLN. In line 4, airway obstruction is again present in addition to a low FEV_1, yet 6% had normal $FEF_{25-75\%}$. In line 5, the FEV_1/FVC was significantly reduced indicating larger airway obstruction with normal FEV_3/FVC and normal FVC, yet 56% had normal $FEF_{25-75\%}$. In line 6, one might expect from prior biases that the $FEF_{25-75\%}$ might shine in identifying small airway disease in the presence of normal FEV_1/FVC and FVC. However, the $FEF_{25-75\%}$ was normal in 77% of these individuals who had evidence of smaller airway disease disclosed by their reduced FEV_3/FVC (increased $FVC-FEV_3$). Thus over 40% of current smoking population (lines 3-6) with normal FVC but evidence of airway obstruction, have

Table 4-3		Spirometric Patterns in 3,570 NHANES-3 Current Smokers Using 95% Confidence Limits (LLN)						
Line	n	Pattern	FVC	FEV_1	FEV_1/FVC	FEV_3/FVC	$FEF_{25-75\%}$	
							N	A
1	2,403	N	N	N	N	N	99%	1%
2	323	±R, no O	N&A or A& N		N	N	80%	20%
3	268	+O	N	N	A	A	42%	58%
4	170	+O	N	A	A	A	6%	94%
5	126	+O, lg	N	A or N	A	N	56%	44%
6	119	+O, sm	N	A or N	N	A	77%	23%
7	118	+O, ±R	A	A	A&A, A&N, or N&A		6%	94%
8	43	Others	A or N	A or N	A or N	A or N	53%	47%

n = number of subjects, Red = probable false positive, Blue = probable false negative (A = abnormal or below LLN, N = normal, O = obstruction, R = restriction, lg = predominantly larger airways, sm = predominantly smaller airways, + = condition present, ± = condition may be present)

$FEF_{25-75\%}$ values above the proper LLN. Further, $FEF_{25-75\%}$ values between 65% and 80% of mean predicted in adults are never below the LLN. As one might suspect, the false negative $FEF_{25-75\%}$ findings tend to be more likely in older individuals where the proper LLN for $FEF_{25-75\%}$ is often close to zero.

Others

Lines 7 and 8 other of the 3,570 current smokers with abnormal spirometry requiring further investigation to identify their problems.

Conclusion

Thus, it should be evident from this large smoking population of three ethnicities and both genders from 20 to 79 years of age that the $FEF_{25-75\%}$ measurement is often falsely positive and often falsely negative, due in large part to its inherent high variability. It also represents differing portions of expiratory flow depending on the absence or severity of airway obstruction. Fortunately, there is a good spirometric measure which has been underutilized in the past. The FEV_3/FVC (or $1\text{-}FEV_3/FVC$) is always at the end of a forced expiration, whether there is a small or large volume exhaled after 3 seconds. It is easy to measure. Reference values are available. It should be routinely reported and interpreted.

HOW BEST TO REPORT AND INTERPRET SPIROMETRY VALUES

Included in the report, besides laboratory identification, locale, and date, should be the name, age or birth date and ethnicity as given by the patient; complaint or reason for the test, and name of the requesting physician; measured shoeless height (or arms span when necessary) and measured unencumbered weight and the source(s) of the predicting equations used in the interpretations.

Traditional Tabular Format

A traditional tabular format for presenting spirometric data is: (A) The left hand column gives mean predicted values for measurements of patients of that age, height, gender and ethnicity. (B) The second column gives actual best values for each measurement recorded. (C) The third column gives percentage of predicted, i.e., 100 times actual/predicted. Sometimes values below 80% are colored or emboldened; at other times values below the 95% confidence limits are asterisked or emboldened. Emboldening values below the 95% confidence limits rather than below 80% of predicted is far preferable.

If an aerosolized bronchodilator was administered, column B is likely to be split so that the left side has best pre-BD values and right side has best post-BD values. Rarely there may be another column which gives percentage (or absolute) changes between pre-BD and post-BD values. Some laboratories list all (or even more) of the measures listed in tables 4-1 and 4-2, but omit IC and ERV, which are useful in assessing the effect of obesity. Some laboratories give samples of time versus volume or volume versus flow tracings alone or samples of best pre-BD and post-BD tracings.

Traditional Interpretation

The interpreting laboratory physician should ultimately comment on the quality of the test, especially if there were problems in language communication, cooperation, if patient was unable to perform well due to fatigue, chest pain or other cause, if the patient had received aerosolized bronchodilators within the few hours before laboratory BD testing, or if the patient's age or height were outside the limits of the population from which the predicting equations were derived.

The interpreting laboratory physician typically selects the few values that the physician considers important and states that they are normal, borderline abnormal or clearly abnormal. There is a strong consensus that the presence or absence of obstruction is dependent on the $\%FEV_1/FVC$ and that the degree of obstruction is dependent on comparing the actual FEV_1 to the mean predicted FEV_1. The latest ATS/ERS guidelines[15] suggest that if the $\%FEV_1/FVC$ is above the 95% confidence limits and the FEV_1 is above 80% of mean predicted, airway obstruction is not present. The guidelines[15] suggest that if the $\%FEV_1/FVC$ is below the 95% confidence limits and the FEV_1 is above 80% or 100% of mean predicted, that combination may not be airway obstruction but a "physiological variant." Data of Hyatt et al.[16] suggest that most individuals with this combination have mild obstructive airway disease. Experience here agrees with that conclusion. If the $\%FEV_1/FVC$ is below the 95% confidence limit, the ATS/ERS recommends grading the severity of obstruction on the relationship of actual FEV_1 to predicted FEV_1 as follows: 70-80%—mild; 60-69%—moderate; 50-59%—moderately severe; 35-49%—severe and less than 35%—very severe.[15] Fortunately, the last ATS/ERS committee report does not recommend use of the $FEF_{25-75\%}$ to diagnose small airways disease. Despite this, it still is a custom of some physicians to interpret $FEF_{25-75\%}$ values below 80% of mean predicted as abnormal or borderline or suggestive or indicative of small airways disease. For a multitude of reasons, I believe these $FFF_{25-75\%}$ interpretations are, more often than not, flawed and misleading.

Some physicians interpret the combination of a reduced FVC and entirely normal FEV_1/FVC as indicating restrictive lung disease, even when the TLC has not been measured. I agree with the ATS/ERS statement[15] that restriction is possible or even likely in such cases, but that a definitive diagnosis should not be made in the absence of TLC measurement.

Finally, the interpretation of lung function is incomplete if spirometry alone has been performed. Further information can be obtained from lung volume measurements and especially from single-breath measurement of diffusing capacity of the lung for carbon monoxide (DLCO) also known as transfer factor of the lung for carbon monoxide (TLCO), which measurements include those of the effective alveolar volume (VA') by an accompanying inert relatively insoluble gas. Additional information is obtainable from non-invasive oximetry, measurements of arterial blood gas and pH, ventilation, end-tidal or mixed-expired CO_2 and O_2 and exercise testing.[3]

GOLD Interpretation

The Global Initiative for Chronic Obstructive Lung Disease (GOLD)[17] for many years has recommended that the diagnosis of COPD should be entertained or made if the baseline %FEV_1/FVC is 70% or less and the FEV_1 is less than 80% of mean predicted, regardless of the age or symptoms of that individual. More recently, it modified these criteria by recommending that COPD can be diagnosed, regardless of age or percent of predicted FEV_1, if the post-aerosolized bronchodilator %FEV1/FVC is 70% or less.[17] Despite the good intentions, expertise and international composition of this organization, many other investigators and committees, for several reasons, believe these recommendations are incorrect and should be abandoned.[13-15,18-20] Some reasons follow.

First, figure 4-22 shows that many younger individuals with %FEV_1/FVC above 70% (blue) clearly are well below the 95% confidence limits calculated from the well-accepted reference population equations of Hankinson et al.[8] They are false negatives if one had used the GOLD criteria. These individuals have airway obstruction, whether due to asthma, chronic bronchitis or some other disorders *and should not be falsely classified as normal.*

Second, many older individuals have %FEV_1/FVC that are below 70% (black). They are false positives, since their values are well above the 95% confidence limits for their age and size. To label such individuals using the GOLD criterion as "obstructive lung disease" and to recommend or prescribe drugs for such individuals, regardless of their symptoms or lack of symptoms, seems unwise, unnecessary and in some cases dangerous. Figure 4-23 shows the increasing number of never-smokers classified by ethnicity and gender *who would be falsely identified as "abnormal" if the then current GOLD criterion were utilized.*

Third, the more recently revised GOLD requirement and emphasis on using post-BD rather than pre-BD values[17] makes spirometry more time-consuming and complicated, and will miss a number of individuals who may have ordinary or occupational asthma and would benefit from further evaluation and treatment.

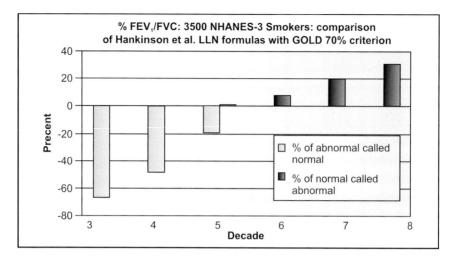

Figure 4-22 Comparison of 3,500 current-smoking NHANES-3 subjects showing the large percentages (in blue) of individuals with "abnormal" %FEV$_1$/FVC by Hankinson et al.[8] reference equations which are called "normal" using %FEV$_1$/FVC greater than 70% (GOLD criterion) and large percentage of individuals with "normal" %FEV$_1$/FVC by Hankinson et al. reference equations which are called "abnormal" using GOLD criterion.[17]

A Better Tabular Format for Interpretation

An improved tabular way (Table 4-4) is to present spirometric data for evidence of airway obstruction using the following format:

- The left hand column identifies the measurements and units.
- The next column presents mean predicted values for measurements of patients of that age, height, gender, and ethnicity.
- The next column presents the upper and/or lower limits of normal (1.645 times SEE, Syx or RSD) values for each predicted value.
- The next column presents several trials or the single best before B-D values for each measurement recorded.
- If an aerosolized bronchodilator was administered, the next column presents several trials or the single best after B-D values.
- Values which are beyond the normal range can be underlined or asterisked. Percent of predicted values are not given.
- For spirometry, only the measures listed in table 4-1 are used.

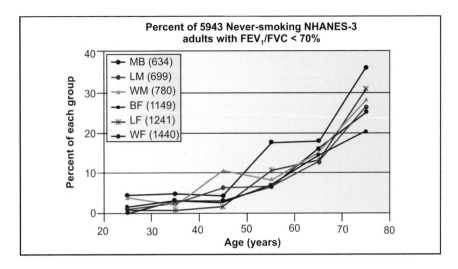

Figure 4-23 Percentage of apparently healthy never-smoking NHANES-3 adults, by decade, gender and ethnicity, who would be considered "abnormal" using GOLD criteria of %FEV$_1$/FVC below 70%.[17]

The interpreter can easily note which values are above or below 95% limits of normal.[14,15] The interpreter also has access to all tracings including pre-BD and post-BD tests (can be printed on the form) to evaluate the patient's ability to cooperate and the consistency and quality of the tracings. By reviewing 1-FEV$_3$/FVC values the interpreter can evaluate small airways function or dysfunction, in case it differs from larger airways function or dysfunction.

If the interpreter feels there is airway obstruction he/she can decide if it is possible, borderline, trivial, minimal, mild, moderate, moderately severe, severe or very severe based on the totality of information present. If other lung volume data are available, the interpreter can grade if there is a ventilatory defect on the basis of actual FEV$_1$ to predicted FEV$_1$, the ventilatory defect's overall severity and attempt to divide the ventilatory defect into obstructive and restrictive components, each with its degree of severity. The interpretation of bronchodilator effect will be discussed in the next chapter.

Another Better Interpretation Method: Grades

The author believes that it often gives a false impression or interpretation of "normalcy" to consider that everyone above the 95% confidence limit for %FEV$_1$/FVC does not have evidence for airway obstruction.[21] There is no question that as a

Table 4-4 Suggested (partial) Format for Reports				
Identifying	Data			
Measurement, units	Mean predicted	LLN/ULN	Before BD	After BD
Volumes				
SVC, L	3.31	2.67	1.56	
FVC, L	3.31	2.67	1.56	1.74
IC, L	2.28		1.11	1.36
ERV, L	1.03		0.45	0.38
Flows				
FEV$_1$, L, trial 1	2.70	2.16	0.85	1.01
FEV$_1$, L, trial 2	"	"	0.88	1.01
FEV$_1$, L, trial 3	"	"	0.87	0.96
FEV$_1$/FVC, %	81%	72%	56%	
FEV$_3$, L, trial 1	3.15	2.56	1.20	1.38
FEV$_3$, L, trial 2	"	"	1.21	1.36
FEV$_3$, L, trial 3	"	"	1.21	1.32
1-FEV$_3$/FVC,%	5.0%	10.5%	22.4%	

group, cigarette smokers have significantly lower %FEV$_1$/FVC than never-smokers.[21] Can we transfer this knowledge to the individual smoker?

Consider a somewhat parallel consideration in grade or intermediate school. Some schools or teachers grade only as satisfactory or unsatisfactory; others grade with letter: A, B, C, D, E, F. There is no inherent reason why airway function cannot also be similarly graded.[21] Suggestions are given in table 4-5. One can hope that current smokers would be better influenced by their physicians and other health professionals or counselors to stop smoking after telling the patient that their airway function was graded as a D or E rather than telling them their airway function was normal or within normal limits. A grade of D or especially a grade of E or F would also warrant a more complete clinical evaluation including history and physical and measurement of carbon monoxide diffusing capacity (DLCO) also identified as the CO transfer factor (TLCO) and lung volumes.

Another Better Interpretation Method to Consider: Lung Age

There is also a reasonable amount of variability in spirometric measures of never-smoking populations without recognized asthma. Part of this variability is inherent; other variability may be due to prior infections; exposure to second-hand smoke

Table 4-5	Grading of %FEV$_1$/FVC and %FEV$_1$/FEV$_6$ for Airway Obstruction Using Predicted and Actual Values[21]		
Actual %FEV$_1$/FVC minus predicted %FEV$_1$/FVC	Actual %FEV$_1$/FEV$_6$ minus predicted %FEV$_1$/FEV$_6$	Grade	Comment
> +6%	> +8%	A	Well above average
+6 to +3%	+8 to +4%	B	Above average
+3% to –3%	+4% to –4%	C	Average
–3 to –6%	–4% to –8%	D	Below average
–6 % to –9%	–8% to –12%	E	Much below average
< –9%	< –12%	F	Abnormal; grade from mild to very severe

or a variety of recognized or unrecognized noxious fumes, particles, pollens or chemicals; or secondary to unrecognized cardiovascular or other system disease. "Reference" populations, from whom reference equations are derived, always includes volunteers who may predominantly be above average in health as well as other individuals with unrecognized illnesses.

It is apparent that ratios of FEV$_1$/FVC or FEV$_1$/FEV$_6$ gradually decrease with advancing age in normal populations. The average FEV$_1$/FVC and FEV$_1$/FEV$_6$ ratios also decrease with increasing airway obstruction. As shown in figure 4-24, in the large NHANES-3 population, the current-smokers' %FEV$_1$/FVC and %FEV$_1$/FEV$_6$ of every decade of age were consistently below those of never-smokers of the same decades.[21] Despite population variability, when %FEV$_1$/FVC or %FEV$_1$/FEV$_6$ were reduced below that expected for a given age, gender and size that was evidence of airway obstruction. In attempting to quantify the increase in lung age due to smoking we compared young never-smokers to older current-smokers, and found that average lung age increased by 3 years for every 1% decrease in %FEV$_1$/FVC below mean predicted and that average lung age increased by 4 years for every 1% decrease in %FEV$_1$/FEV$_6$ below mean predicted. We therefore translated %FEV$_1$/FVC and %FEV$_1$/FEV$_6$ values for over 5,800 NHANES-3 never-smokers and 3,500 current smokers of both genders and three ethnicities into lung ages.[21]

In 1985, Morris and Temple[22] introduced the concept of increased lung age due to smoking. They derived and publishing formulas which included FEV$_1$ or FVC plus age, height and gender to calculate the equivalent lung age of a group of smokers compared to never-smokers. In figure 4-25, Plot A shows the lung age values calculated from the Morris and Temple equations for the white NHANES-3 population.

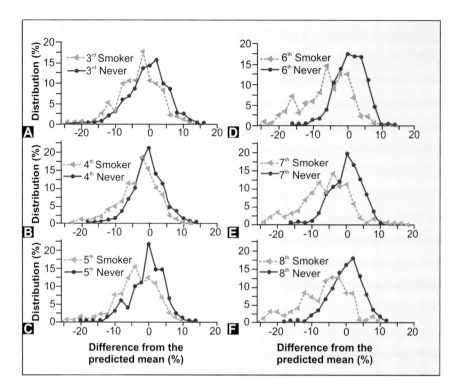

Figure 4-24 Severity of airflow obstruction measured by %FEV$_1$/FVC over six decades of age for over 3,500 NHANES-3 current-smokers and 5,800 NHANES-3 never-smokers. Percentage deviations grouped every 2% from mean predicted values of never-smokers are graphed. Differences between never- and current-smokers increase until the 6th decade and then apparently stabilize (The NHANES-3 population did not include any subjects with very severe airway obstruction).

   Although individual lung ages of each population varied considerably, the majority of individual smoker's lung ages increased rapidly above their actual ages, especially until they reached their 6th decade (age 50–59). In figure 4-25, Plot B, C. and D compares changes in mean lung age from mean actual age in each ethnic, group using our formula. Thereafter the 20–25 year differences between actual age and lung age did not increase except in the Latin group. The lack of further increase in recorded airway obstruction may have been due to cardiovascular, respiratory, and malignancy-associated mortality and morbidity associated with long-term smoking which deleted the potential population sample in the 6th through 8th decades. No participants in the NHANES-3 survey had very severe obstructive airways disease.[21] Thus, older potential NHANES-3 current-smokers may have been confined and unable to participate due to the severity of their obstructive airways disease.

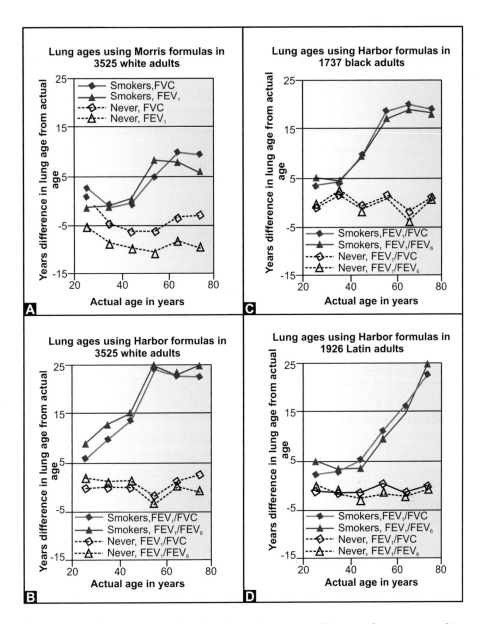

Figure 4-25 Comparisons, by decade, of never-smoking and current-smoking NHANES-3 populations of Morris and Temple lung age equations in white adults (Plot A) with Harbor lung age equations in white, black and Latin populations (Plots B, C and D). New equations are: for every 1% decrease from predicted FEV_1/FVC, lung age increases by 3 years; for every 1% decrease from predicted FEV_1/FEV_6, lung age increases by 4 years.

As with the use of grades, informing smoking patients that their lung ages calculated from spirometry were higher than their actual age by 10 or more years (when in their earlier decades) or by 20 or more years in their middle age should reinforce other efforts by their health professionals to induce them to join a program to stop smoking. If they are never-smokers, further inquiry into their respiratory, occupational or recreational status may be useful in uncovering asthma, occupational lung disease or over-exposure to noxious particulates in their living or working environments.

Interpreting 1-FEV_3/FVC or FEV_3/FVC

Not surprisingly, the FEV_1/FVC and FEV_3/FVC values in populations are highly correlated. It seems sensible to include interpretation of the FEV_3/FVC in deciding whether or not a subject has airway obstruction.[12,23,24] Although it is reasonable to interpret values of FEV_3/FVC below the 95% confidence limit as evidence of smaller airways obstruction, there has not been adequate investigation to use the FEV_3/FVC measurement to quantify airway obstruction. Thus, it can be used diagnostically, but perhaps not to quantify degree of airway obstruction. With further experience, it may ultimately help discriminate between airway obstructions which are asthmatic and that which are emphysematous.

COMPARATIVE ANALYSES OF SELECTED SPIROMETRIC REFERENCE EQUATIONS

Now that we are aware of the wide scatter of differences in individuals in any single series, it is not surprising that there are differences in mean values and variability for predicted reference equations in different reported series. It is often recommended that each laboratory select a number of normal individuals in their area, measure their spirometric values and ascertain how well they fit one or more predicting equations. That may be optimal but it is time consuming, rarely practical and requires developing consent forms and obtaining permission from a Human Subjects Committee. Following are shown the calculated values derived from reference equations for a given gender, age, and height for a number of spirometric variables in a large number of series of never-smoking, apparently normal adults. We felt it instructive and necessary to examine these differences or similarities between series not only for mean ages and heights but also over a wider range of ages and heights.

FEV_1 Values for White Men

First, the FEV_1, FVC and %FEV_1/FVC formulas (found in APPENDIX) from series of never-smoking men and women will be presented and analyzed, as these formulas are frequently used as reference equations and patient values are commonly compared to these reference values and interpreted clinically (Table 4-6 and Figure 4-26). In the next four tables and figures, 8 equations are identified by the first letter of the first authors' last name, the letter "J" identifies the linear equations derived by JE Hansen from NHANES-3 data and the letter "S" identifies the SHIP equations.[8,24-32] Populations identified by the series authors as "white" or "Caucasian" from North America and Europe were chosen to minimize differences that might be related to ethnicity or nutrition. Each of the 10 equations was used to calculate predicted values for each of nine conditions (30, 50, and 70 years at heights of 165, 175, and 185 cm).

This range of heights included 87% of the population of the white NHANES-3 never-smokers between ages 20 and 80 years. Of that population, only 4% were shorter and 9% were taller. This height range also included 75% of the Latin men and 85% of the black men.

Note the reasonably parallel but considerable differences between the reference equation values in each group of ten shown in figure 4-26. For each of the nine conditions, the arithmetic and absolute differences of each calculated value from the mean values of each of the nine conditions were derived. These were then summed. Rank orders of these series were assigned giving equal weight to the arithmetic and absolute differences from the mean values at each of the nine conditions related to age and height. The equation with the lowest deviations from the means of the nine conditions was identified as 1; that with the highest deviations was identified as 10.

Table 4-6	The FEV$_1$ Values for White Men: Difference from the Mean Predicted Values in Liters Using Ten Reference Equations at Ages 30, 50, and 70 years and Heights of 185, 175, and 165 cm				
Initial	First author	Locale	Mean arithmetic difference (L)	Mean absolute difference (L)	Overall rank
C	Crapo	Utah (USA)	+0.076	0.092	4
G	Gutierrez	Canada	+0.134	0.134	5
H	Hankinson	USA	−0.006	0.045	2
J	J Hansen	USA	−0.005	0.035	1
K	Knudson	Arizona (USA)	−0.096	0.148	7
M	Miller	Great Britain	−0.206	0.206	10
P	Paoletti	Italy	−0.065	0.065	3
Q	Quanjer	Europe	−0.174	0.174	8
R	Roca	Mediterranean	+0.201	0.201	9
S	SHIP authors	Germany	+0.142	0.142	6

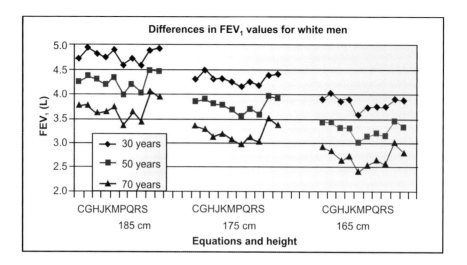

Figure 4-26 Predicted FEV$_1$ values for white men using 10 reference equations. The results depict values at ages 30, 50, and 70 years of age and 185, 175, and 165 cm of height. The formulas used, from left to right are from Crapo (C), Gutierrez (G), Hankinson (H), J Hansen (J), Knudson (K), Miller (M), Paoletti (P), Quanjer (Q), Roca (R) and SHIP (S) authors and their colleagues. The average values may not necessarily be best. One can note, for example, that the Knudson values are well above average for taller individuals but well below average for shorter individuals, while Roca and SHIP values tend to always be above average.

Three of the five North American series and three of the five European series were below the mean values while two of the five North American series and two of the five European series were above the mean values (Table 4-6). The extremes of values at any given height and age ranged 340–670 mL, averaging 500 mL. The percentage of maximal differences at all nine conditions ranged 8–25%. The absolute and percentage differences were wider at 165 and 185 cm whereas the widest percentage differences were at age 70. The European series differed more from each other than the North American series. Formula results varied more widely as age or height differed from the median values of 50 years and 175 cm. Thus, one should be more cautious in interpreting pulmonary function tests at the extremes. There is no certainty that the mean values of the ten series at any one height and age are the best to use, but the overall mean FEV$_1$ values are likely reasonable for white men in North America and Europe. It is also likely, that self-identified so-called "white" populations may vary considerably within a single country and from one continent to the other.

FVC Values for White Men

Figure 4-27 and table 4-7 are for FVC from the same series for white men used in the prior section. In this case, four of the North American and three of the European series were above the overall mean values. The maximal percentage of differences for the nine conditions ranged between 10% and 27% with an average maximal difference of 16%.

FEV$_1$ Values for White Women

In a similar way, figure 4-28 and table 4-8 present values of FEV$_1$ calculated from the same series[8,24-32] as in table 4-6 and figure 4-26. The height range of 150-170 cm includes over 80% of the black and white women and 65% of the Latin women. Values between series for the same age and height may vary as much as 500 mL, i.e., about 20%. Two of the five American series and three of the five European series were below the overall mean values. As with the men, there are somewhat lesser divergences from the overall means with the North American series.

FVC Values for White Women

Figure 4-29 and table 4-9 present FVC values for white women at 30–70 years and 150–170 cm in height. Although the absolute differences between FVC values are wider than those for FEV$_1$ in women and less than those for men, the percentage spread is over 30%. The simple linear equations of JE Hansen[32] found in the appendix are closest to the mean values of the ten different series.

%FEV$_1$/FVC for White Men

Following are a figure and table with values for %FEV$_1$/FVC from several series for white men (Figure 4-30 and Table 4-10). The first four series[8,24,25,32] were selected because equations were available for both FEV$_1$/FVC directly and those some values could be derived independently from separate predicting equations for FEV$_1$ and FVC. Values were identified and selected in the following ways: c, g, h, and j identify values from direct single equations; C, G, H, and J identify values derived from dividing the values from each series; FEV$_1$ values by the same series; FVC values shown in figures 4-26 and 4-27. The v and V values are previously published linear equations from NHANES-3 data, each derived using predicted FVC rather than actual height; v was derived only from white men;[12] V was a single equation derived from three ethnicities and two genders.[12] The percentage differences in FEV$_1$/FVC between series (maximum of 5%) were much less than the percentage differences found when calculating absolute FVC and FEV$_1$ for the same ages and heights.

Note that divergences are greater in shorter and older men. Sometimes the differences between the direct single equations and combination of two equations

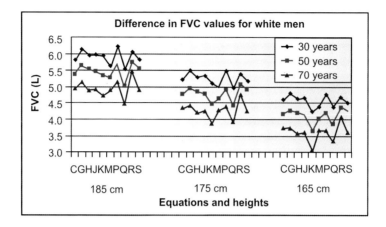

Figure 4-27 Differences in FVC values for white men at three ages and three heights. Format and abbreviations are identical to those of Figure 4-26.

Table 4-7	The FVC Values for White Men. Difference from the Mean Predicted Values in Liters Using Ten Reference Equations at Ages 30, 50, and 70 years and Heights of 185, 175, and 165 cm				
Initial	First author	Locale	Mean arithmetic difference (L)	Mean absolute difference (L)	Overall rank
C	Crapo	Utah (USA)	+0.010	0.057	2
G	Gutierrez	Canada	+0.182	0.182	7
H	Hankinson	USA	+0.030	0.061	4
J	J Hansen	USA	+0.026	0.033	1
K	Knudson	Arizona (USA)	−0.272	0.280	8
M	Miller	Great Britain	−0.120	0.135	5
P	Paoletti	Italy	+0.168	0.168	6
Q	Quanjer	Europe	−0.330	0.330	10
R	Roca	Mediterranean	+0.305	0.305	9
S	SHIP authors	Germany	+0.002	0.075	3

(FEV_1 and FVC) differ by more than one percent. The Crapo et al. values may be elevated because lower gas density at higher altitude increases the FEV_1 but not the FVC. The J and j values are closest to the overall mean values.

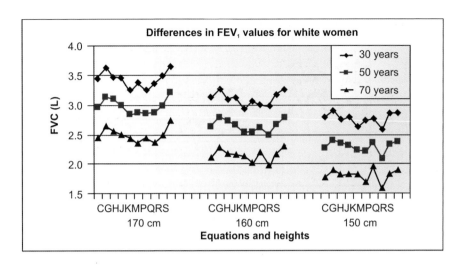

Figure 4-28 Predicted FEV$_1$ values for white women using 10 reference equations. The results depict values at ages 30, 50, and 70 years of age and 170, 160, and 150 cm of height. For further information please see the legend for Figure 4-26.

Table 4-8	The FEV$_1$ Values for White Women. Differences from the Mean Predicted Values in Liters Using Ten Reference Equations at Ages 30, 50, and 70 years and Heights of 170, 160, and 150 cm			
Initial	First author	Locale	Mean arithmetic difference (L)	Mean absolute difference (L)	Overall rank
C	Crapo	Utah (USA)	−0.011	0.029	2
G	Gutierrez	Canada	+0.139	0.139	8
H	Hankinson	USA	+0.037	0.044	4
J	J Hansen	USA	+0.015	0.015	1
K	Knudson	Arizona (USA)	−0.096	0.099	7
M	Miller	Great Britain	−0.090	0.090	6
P	Paoletti	Italy	−0.024	0.086	5
Q	Quanjer	Europe	−0.160	0.160	10
R	Roca	Mediterranean	+0.035	0.037	3
S	SHIP authors	Germany	+0.158	0.158	9

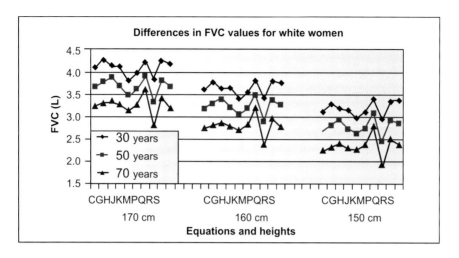

Figure 4-29 Predicted FVC values for white women using 10 reference equations. The results depict values at ages 30, 50, and 70 years of age and 170, 160, and 150 cm of height. For further information please see the legend for Figure 4-26.

Table 4-9		The FVC Values for White Women. Difference from the Mean Predicted Values in Liters Using Ten Reference Equations at Ages 30, 50, and 70 years and Heights of 170, 160, and 150 cm			
Initial	First author	Locale	Mean arithmetic difference (L)	Mean absolute difference (L)	Overall rank
C	Crapo	Utah (USA)	−0.050	0.052	3
G	Gutierrez	Canada	+0.069	0.075	5
H	Hankinson	USA	+0.084	0.086	6
J	JE Hansen	USA	−0.013	0.024	1
K	Knudson	Arizona (USA)	−0.174	0.174	8
M	Miller	Great Britain	−0.042	0.056	2
P	Paoletti	Italy	+0.277	0.277	9
Q	Quanjer	Europe	−0.338	0.338	10
R	Roca	Mediterranean	+0.148	0.148	7
S	SHIP authors	Germany	+0.041	0.069	4

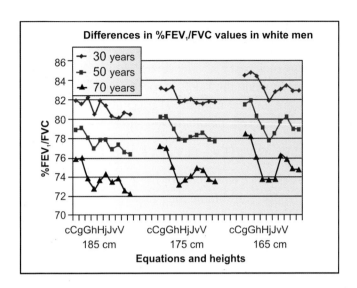

Figure 4-30 Differences in %FEV$_1$/FVC values for white men at three ages and three heights from 10 sets of equations. The c, g, h, and j use direct %FEV$_1$/FVC equations. The C, G, H, and J each use two equations, i.e., the ratio of the FEV$_1$ equation values to the FVC equation values. The v and V use FVC values rather than height. See text for further explanation.

Table 4-10	The %FEV$_1$/FVC Values for White Men. Difference from the Mean Predicted Values in Percent Using Reference Equations at Ages 30, 50, and 70 years and Heights of 185, 175, and 165 cm				
Initial	First author	Type	Mean arithmetic difference (%)	Mean absolute difference (%)	Overall rank
c	Crapo	Single	+1.67	1.67	9
C	Crapo	FEV$_1$ and FVC	+1.69	1.69	10
g	Gutierrez	Single	+0.65	0.65	4
G	Gutierrez	FEV$_1$ and FVC	−0.84	0.84	6
h	Hankinson	Single	−0.74	0.97	7
H	Hankinson	FEV$_1$ and FVC	−0.43	0.65	3
j	JE Hansen	Single	−0.22	0.45	2
J	JE Hansen	FEV$_1$ and FVC	−0.11	0.31	1
v	JE Hansen	Using FVC	−0.75	0.75	5
V	JE Hansen	Using FVC	−0.91	0.91	8

%FEV₁/FVC Values for White Women

Figure 4-31 and table 4-11 show the values of $\%FEV_1/FVC$ for white women of the same ages as for white men.[8,12,24,25,32] The single $\%FEV_1/FVC$ equation of Gutierrez is closest to the average while the values derived from the pair of FEV_1 and FVC Gutierrez equations are furthest from the average of all 10 sets of equations. The widest range of differences is 7%, found in older and shorter women.

FEV₃/FEV₆, FEV₁/FEV₆, FEV₃/FEV₆, FEV₃/FVC and 1-FEV₃/FVC

There are not many reference equations for these measurements. Those available are given in the Appendix. The volume measures (FEV_3, FEV_6) are ethnic, gender, age and height specific; ratio measures derived by us are dependent only on size of the FVC. Note that if the predicted or actual value for FEV_3/FVC is 0.92 or 92%, the actual or predicted value for $1\text{-}FEV_3/FVC$ would be 0.08 or 8%.

Figures 4-32 and 4-33 show the relationship between all these ratios and the FVC in thousands of never-smoking men and women. Three ethnicities were combined to increase the data size. These plots are remarkably linear from age 18 to 78 years, except for likely flattening of the curves as one goes from older to younger ages near age 22-20 in the FEV_6/FVC, FEV_3/FEV_6 and FEV_3/FVC ratios. Table 4-12 gives the slopes and intercepts.

SELECTION OF REFERENCE EQUATIONS

For Blacks, Latins, and Whites

Each of the reference equations published in the Appendix have merit. However, if a laboratory decides to change to new reference equations, some confusion may result, as interpretations are somewhat dependent on the reference equations used. As one can see in the figures of this chapter, the differences between equations occur not only at the higher and lower heights and ages but also at median heights and ages.

The differences between the values of different series of volume equations (FVC, FEV_1, FEV_3 and FEV_6) have a wider scatter than do those between series of ratios (FEV_1/FVC, FEV_1/FEV_6, FEV_3/FVC, FEV_3/FEV_6). Table 4-13 shows the average absolute differences compared to the mean values of each series at 50 years of age and 175 cm for men and 160 cm for women. It is important to note in this table that the differences between predicting equations for the ratios of $\%FEV_1/FVC$ are 3-4 times less than those for the volume equations of FEV_1 and FVC. The same is true if we were to use any volume to volume ratio and compare it to the absolute values of the equations from which the ratio is derived. This reduced scatter in reference equations of ratios implies that we can rely more on the ratios that define and sometime quantify obstruction than on the volumes that may define and quantify

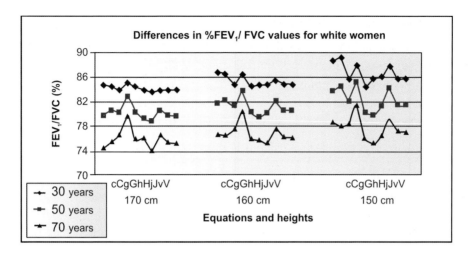

Figure 4-31 Differences in %FEV$_1$/FVC values for white women at three ages and three heights from 10 sets of equations. The c, g, h, and j use direct %FEV$_1$/FVC equations. The C, G, H, and J each use two equations, i.e., the ratio of the FEV$_1$ equation values to the FVC equation values. The v and V use FVC values rather than height. See text for further explanation.

Table 4-11	The %FEV$_1$/FVC Values for White Women. Difference from the Mean Predicted Values in Percent Using Reference Equations at Ages 30, 50, and 70 years and Heights of 170, 160, and 150 cm				
Initial	First author	Type	Mean arithmetic difference (%)	Mean absolute difference (%)	Overall rank
c	Crapo	Single	+0.51	0.96	6
C	Crapo	FEV$_1$ and FVC	+0.79	0.94	5
g	Gutierrez	Single	+0.01	0.48	1
G	Gutierrez	FEV$_1$ and FVC	+2.45	2.45	10
h	Hankinson	Single	−0.97	1.04	7
H	Hankinson	FEV$_1$ and FVC	−1.14	1.16	9
j	JE Hansen	Single	−1.09	1.09	8
J	JE Hansen	FEV$_1$ and FVC	+0.72	0.81	4
v	JE Hansen	Using FVC	−0.62	0.62	2
V	JE Hansen	Using FVC	−0.64	0.64	3

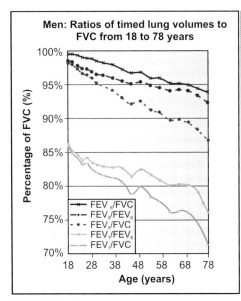

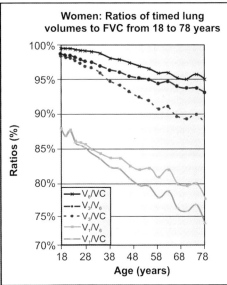

Figure 4-32 Changes of several spirometric ratios to the highest FVC at any age, usually ages 18–22 years in men. Data of all three ethnicities are combined into two year groupings from age 18 to 78 years. The highest average FVC measured for each ethnicity in age group is considered to be 100%. Considering the diversity of the population, the slopes are quite linear. The slopes of FEV_6/FVC, FEV_3/FEV_6 and FEV_3/FVC appear to be slightly less steep between 18 and 22 years. For men, the size of subjects in each ethnic and age group averaged 45, but ranged in size from 5 to 129 subjects, lowest in number at older ages.

Figure 4-33 Changes of several spirometric ratios to the highest FVC at any age, usually ages 18–22 years, in women. Data of all three ethnicities are combined into two year groupings ages 18–78 years. The highest average FVC measured for each ethnicity in age group is considered to be 100%. Considering the diversity of the population, the slopes are quite linear. The slopes of FEV_6/FVC, FEV_3/FEV_6 and FEV_3/FVC appear to be slightly less steep between 18 and 22 years. For women, the size of each ethnic and age group averaged 74, but ranges in size from 15 to 133 subjects, with numbers less dependent on age.

restriction. In other words, there is more population variability in any one or more volumes than in the ratios of one volume to another volume.

There is another factor to consider in using the ratio of $\%FEV_1/FVC$. We realize that nearly all spirometric volume (FEV_1, FEV_3, FEV_6, FVC) predicting equations consist of a constant plus a variable multiplied times height plus another variable multiplied times age. The same is true of most but not all of direct $\%FEV_1/FVC$

Table 4-12	Slopes and Intercepts for Timed Lung Volume Ratios Age 18–78 years			
	Men		Women	
Ratio	Slopes/decade	Intercepts	Slopes/decade	Intercepts
FEV_6/FVC	0.97%	102%	0.94%	101%
FEV_3/FEV_6	0.89%	100%	0.76%	100%
FEV_3/FVC	1.79%	101%	1.63%	102%
FEV_1/FEV_6	1.22%	87%	1.29%	88%
FEV_1/FVC	1.98%	88%	2.00%	89%

Table 4-13	Comparing Variability Between Predicting Equations at 50 years of Age and 75 cm Height for Men and 160 cm Height for Women		
Gender, measure, unit	Average absolute differences from mean	Average mean	Average difference/ Average mean
Men, FEV_1, L	0.163 L	4.759 L	3.43%
Women, FEV_1, L	0.130 L	3.246 L	4.00%
Men, FVC, L	0.124 L	3.763 L	3.30%
Women, FVC, L	0.086 L	2.635 L	3.26%
Men, FEV_1/FVC, %	0.89%	78.52%	1.13%
Women, FEV_1/FVC, %	0.70%	80.12%	0.87%

equations. The equations of Hankinson et al.[8] are exceptions in that the constant and age are used in their direct %FEV_1/FVC predicting equations, but height or FVC are not. We recognized and reported that the relatively small differences in predicting equations for three ethnicities and the two genders was primarily due to the differences in FVC values for the same height in these differing ethnicities and genders. Therefore, some of our equations for %FEV_1/FVC, %FEV_1/FVC, %FEV_3/FVC and FEV_3/FEV_6 are valid for all genders and three (or probably more) ethnicities and use a constant, a variable times age and a variable times actual or predicted FVC.[12,23]

Other than the two direct %FEV_1/FVC equations of Hankinson et al.[8] used in tables 4-10 and 4-11, the 18 predicting equations[24-32] reveal that the differences of 20 cm in height result in an average difference between taller (185 cm for men and 170 cm for women) in %FEV_1/FVC are 2.8%, 2.4% and 2.2% less for taller than shorter adults at ages 30, 50, and 70 years, respectively. This suggests that using the paired FEV_1 and FVC predicting equations together for %FEV_1/FVC is preferable to using an independent single equation for %FEV_1/FVC which does not include height as a variable.

For Other Ethnicities and Geographic Sites

The task of selecting or modifying reference equations for all populations is an important worldwide challenge. Insufficient information is available for most ethnic/racial/geographic groups. Due to differences in equipment, personnel and techniques, differences in ethnicity seem to be best assessed when the same investigators are measuring two or more ethnic groups simultaneously.

The series presented in this chapter are all from never-smokers, but the influence of second-hand smoke, air contamination or occupational exposures cannot be excluded. In all series included in this chapter, investigators have always attempted to exclude subjects with concurrent musculoskeletal, neurological and cardiovascular disorders or improper tests, but this goal may not always be achieved. It is likely that some of the differences found in ethnic-specific series as compared primarily to European-ethnic (white) populations are due to geographical, nutritional, occupational, air contamination and other differences, not just genetic influences.

The effect of nutrition throughout the lifespan of the test subjects is also likely to be important.[33] Children and youth who grow up in an economically and nutritionally challenged environment may have considerably different lung function as adults than their siblings or cousins who grew up in an environment with ample food and more obesity.

A suggestion is presented here for a reasonable solution for reference equations for ethnicities and geographic sites without reliable reference equations. The author hypothesized that randomly selecting one or two dozen healthy subjects and comparing them to a given reference equation for another ethnicity might be useful. To test this hypothesis, the FEV_1 and FVC values for two series of 12 individuals from the NHANES-3 series of never-smoking healthy black women were randomly selected. When the actual values were compared to the predicted values reference equations of Hankinson et al.[8] in the first series of 12 random subjects, the values were 96.6% and 97.0% of predicted values of FVC and FEV_1, respectively. In the second series of random 12 subjects the respective predicted values were 103.5% and 101.0%. Thus, with 12 random subjects, the values were 1–3.5% in error; with 24 subjects the values were 0.1–2.0% in error. When the values of the 24 black women were used with the white and Latin predicting equations, they averaged 84.8% and 85.1% of the predicted FVC values for white and Latin women, respectively, and 84.1% and 83.9% of the similar predicted FEV1 values. This fits exceptionally well with actual differences among the three ethnicities reported by Hankinson et al.[8] This analysis strongly suggests that measuring the FEV_1 and FVC values from a diverse sample of 12–24 healthy individuals of a single gender, ethnicity and geographic site allows one to quite accurately predict *absolute* reference values of a much larger population at that site for these key spirometric measurements. Ratio values are different. They will differ only slightly or negligibly between populations, in the case of FEV_1/FVC, primarily on the size of the FVC and age of the subject.[32]

SOURCES OF DIFFICULTY

There may be major difficulty in obtaining and interpreting spirometric measures even when the equipment is in order and technicians are well-trained. Communicating with the patient may be difficult. If the patient does not speak the language of the technician, added assistance is necessary. If the patient is weak, confused, or in pain, or sight or hearing-impaired, good cooperation may be impossible. When this is true, recordings should not be discarded even if they are of poor quality as they may contain some useful information when reviewed later by the interpreting physician. Patients on supplemental O_2 should be assessed to ascertain whether or not O_2 can be temporarily discontinued in order to obtain desired tests. Leaks around the mouthpiece and nose are common in ill patients and must be avoided; in some patients special mouthpieces or adaptations may be necessary. Special connections may be necessary in patients with tracheotomies. In patients with spinal deformities or inability to stand, arm span measures should be obtained. In all cases where there are problems in obtaining good quality tracings or when actual height or weight cannot be obtained, the technician should document this so that the interpreting physician is made aware of these circumstances and can comment as necessary to the referring physician.

REFERENCES

1. American Thoracic Society. Standardization of spirometry: 1994 update. *Am J Respir Crit Care Med.* 1995;152:1107-36.
2. Miller MR, Hankinson J, Brusasco V, et al. Standardisation of spirometry. *Eur Respir J.* 2005;26:319-38.
3. Wasserman K, Hansen JE, Sue DY, et al. Principles of Exercise Testing and Interpretation, Including Pathophysiology and Clinical Applications, 4th Edition. Philadelphia, PA: Lippincott Williams and Wilkins; 2004.
4. Gandevia B, Hugh-Jones P. Terminology for measurements of ventilatory capacity. *Thorax.* 1957;1:290-3.
5. Miller WF, Johnson RL Jr, Wu N. relationships between maximal breathing capacity and timed expiratory capacities. *J Appl Physiol.* 1959;14:510-6.
6. Campbell SC. A comparison of the maximum voluntary ventilation with forced expiratory volume in one second: an assessment of subject cooperation. *J Occup Med.* 1982;24:531-3.
7. Ray CS, Sue DY, Bray G, et al. Effects of obesity on respiratory function. *Am Rev Resp Dis.* 1983;128:510-6.

8. Hankinson JL, Odenkranz JR, Fedan KB. Spirometric reference values from a sample of the general U.S. population. *Am J Respir Crit Care Med.* 1999;159(1):179-87.

9. Leuallan EC, Fowler WS. Maximum mid-expiratory flow. *Am Rev Tuberc.* 1955;72:783-800.

10. McFadden ER, Linden DA. A reduction in maximum mid-expiratory flow rate: a spirographic manifestation of small airway disease. *Am J Med.* 1972;52:725-7.

11. Gelb AF, Zamel N. Simplified diagnosis of small airway obstruction. *N Engl J Med.* 1973;288;395-8.

12. Hansen JE, Sun XG, Wasserman K. Discriminating measures and normal values for expiratory obstruction. *Chest.* 2006;129:369-77.

13. Clausen JL. Prediction of Normal Values in Pulmonary Function Testing: Guidelines and Controversies. In: JL Clausen (Ed). New York: Academic Press; 1982.

14. American Thoracic Society. Lung Function Testing: Selection of Reference Values and Interpretative Strategies. *Am Rev Respir Dis.* 1991;144:1202-18.

15. Pelligrino R, Viegi G, Brusasco V, et al. Interpretative strategies for lung function tests. *Eur Respir J.* 2005;26:948-68.

16. Hyatt RE, Cowl CT, Bjoraker JA, et al. Conditions associated with an abnormal nonspecific pattern of pulmonary function tests. *Chest.* 2009;135:419-24.

17. http://www.goldcopd.org/Guidelineitem.asp?l1 = 2&l2 = 1&intld = 2003, accessed May 12, 2010.

18. Roberts SD, Farber MO, Knox KS, et al. FEV1/FVC ratio of 70% misclassifies patients with obstruction at the extremes of age. *Chest.* 2006;130:200-6.

19. Hansen JE, Sun XG, Wasserman K. Spirometric criteria for airway obstruction. Use percentage of FEV1/FVC ratio below the fifth percentile, not < 70%. *Chest.* 2007;131:349-55.

20. Miller MR, Quanjer PH, Swanney MP, et al. Interpreting lung function data using 80 percent of predicted and fixed thresholds misclassifies over 20% of patients. *Chest.* 2010 (in press).

21. Hansen JE, Sun XG, Wasserman K. Calculating odds of low lung function and lung ages for smokers. *Eur Respir J.* 2010;34:776-80.

22. Morris JF, Temple W. Spirometric "lung age" estimation for motivating smoking cessation. *Prev Med.* 1985;14:655-62.

23. Hansen JE, Sun XG, Wasserman K. Ethnic- and sex-free formulae for detection of airway obstruction. *Am J Respir Crit Care.* 2006;174:493-8.

24. Crapo RO, Morris AH, Gardner RM. Reference spirometric values using techniques and equipment that meet ATS recommendations. *Am Rev Respir Dis.* 1981;123:659-64.

25. Gutierrez C, Ghezzo RH, Abboud RT, et al. Reference values of pulmonary function tests for Canadian Caucasians. *Can Respir J.* 2004;11:414-24.

26. Knudson RJ, Lebowitz MD, Holberg CJ. Changes in the normal maximal expiratory flow-volume curve with growth and aging. *Am Rev Respir Dis.* 1983;127:725-34.

27. Miller MR, Grove DM, Pincock AC. Time domain spirogram indices. Their variability and reference values in nonsmokers. *Am Rev Respir Dis.* 1985;132:1041-8.

28. Paoletti P, Pistelli G, Fazzi P, et al. Reference values for vital capacity and flow volume curves from a general population study. *Bull Eur Physiolathol Respir.* 1986;22:451-9.

29. Quanjer PH, Tammeling GJ, Cotes JE, et al. Lung volumes and ventilatory flows. *Eur Respir J.* 1993;6(Suppl. 16):5-40.

30. Roca J, Sanchis J, Agusti-Videl A, et al. Spirometric reference values for a Mediterranean population. *Bull Eur Physiopathol Respir.* 1986;22:451-9.

31. Koch B, Schäper C, Ittermann T, et al. Reference values for lung function testing in adults—results from the study of health in Pomerania (SHIP). *Dtsch Med Wochenschr.* 2009;134:2327-32.

32. Hansen JE. Unpublished observations.

33. Korotzer B, Ong S, Hansen JE. Ethnic differences in pulmonary function in healthy non smoking Asian- and European-Americans. *Am J Respir Crit Care Med.* 2000;161:1101-8.

Assessing Airway Responsiveness in the Laboratory

GENERAL: ASSESSING THE EFFECT OF INTERVENTIONS

Assume that you are told that aerosolizing medication (A) on the throwing arm of some individuals will increase the distance they can throw a given ball. You are asked to test which individuals improve their ability by having the medication sprayed on their throwing arm. You know that some non-athletes can throw the ball 500 cm while some others can throw the ball 5000 cm.

A physician refers five individuals to you for testing the effect of aerosol medications on them. To test the aerosol, you have each one throw the ball satisfactorily three times before (B) the aerosolized medication is sprayed on the throwing arm and three times satisfactorily after (A) the medication is used. But, following tradition and what you have been taught, you do not report the six throws; you consider and report only the longest throw before (B) and after (A) the medication is administered (Table 5-1).

You review these findings and send a report to the referring physician with an interpretation. You use the advice of a committee which recommended that in order to call the medication clinically effective, the throwing distance should increase by both 200 cm and 12%. Therefore, in interpreting the findings you state: Patient 5 responded positively to the medication. Patients 1, 2, 3, and 4 did not clinically respond, but this does not preclude you using the medication.

The physician receiving your report knows that you require 3 throws before and 3 throws after the sprayed medication. Therefore, the referring physician asks you

Table 5-1	Longest Distance in Centimeter Before (B) and After (A) Aerosol Medication on Arm				
Patient	Best B	Best A	Absolute difference	Percent difference	Responder?
1	2000	2150	150	7.5	No
2	600	700	100	16.7	No
3	4000	4400	400	10	No
4	1000	1050	100	5	No
5	2500	3000	500	20	Yes

Table 5-2	All Distances in Centimeter Before (B) and After (A) Aerosol Medication on Arm				
Patient	All (B)	All (A)	Unpaired-1-tailed t-test; $p =$	Rank order test, $p =$	Responder?
1	2000 1950 1980	2010 2150 2120	0.002	0.05	Yes; mild
2	580 600 590	700 680 670	0.0003	0.05	Yes; moderate
3	3950 4000 3080	4400 4350 4300	0.003	0.05	Yes; mild
4	950 1000 980	1050 950 1000	0.51	>0.05	No
5	2500 2460 2480	2950 3000 2900	0.0001	0.05	Yes; moderate

to consider the 6 throws for each individual and not just the best (B) and (A) throws and do a statistical analysis and reinterpretation of the results. One might use the following adjectives to scale for percentage improvements: less than 3% = Trivial or none; 3–6% = minimal and consistent; 6–12% = mild and consistent; 12–24% = moderate and consistent; greater than 24% = marked improvement. In this case, the modifying terms for the five individuals might be: mild, moderate, mild, none, and moderate, respectively.

You do so and find as shown in table 5-2: One patient was a non-responder but the other four were consistent and mild to moderate responders. The referring physician is thankful for your reanalysis.

ASSESSING THE EFFECT OF AEROSOLIZED DRUGS IN THE PULMONARY LABORATORY

Consider that there is a parallel between this theoretical example using distance of throwing a ball (before and after applying aerosolized drug sprayed on the arm) and actual measures of exhaled volumes (before and after applying drugs delivered by aerosol to the lung). One need only substitute volume in milliliter for distance in centimeter.

Historically, but not detailed here, there have been many different suggestions or recommendations as to what should indicate an important or significant, or clinically significant change after administering an aerosolized drug to test for bronchodilation in the laboratory. Now, it is reasonable to ask the origin of the values of 200 mL and 12% recommended by the earlier ATS[1] and more recent ATS/ERS[2] committees. Each committee stated that if both of these criteria were not met, there was "a lack of bronchodilator response".

ASSESSING DATA REPORTED FROM THREE PULMONARY FUNCTION LABORATORIES REGARDING SHORT-TERM VARIABILITY

First, it is clear that measured FEV_1 values in a given individual change somewhat during each day, week or month. Some of that variability is due to the measuring device, which currently requires calibration values of mean volumes to be within 4% ($\pm$ 2%). Some variability is due to intraday changes in patient height or patient maneuver effort, since increased effort may not only increase airflow due to a higher intrathoracic pressure pushing the air out, but may concurrently also decrease airflow due to intrathoracic compression of the airways which increases the resistance. Some variability in an individual is due to airway health or diameter, which can change during mild infections or exposure to allergens, particulates or fumes. However, using the same measuring spirometer on the same patient within a half hour in the same laboratory yields much less variability in values than those found over longer periods of time using different spirometers. Thus, there should be agreement that values obtained within a half hour with the same spirometer in the same environment should be less variable than changes over weeks or months and better represent short-term variability.

Second, let's consider the reported data, statistical analyses and interpretations from three excellent pulmonary function laboratories, each of whom report data in excellent peer reviewed pulmonary journals on a number of individuals with differing degrees of airway obstruction.[3-5] Each used three initial satisfactory forced exhalations meeting ATS standards followed by a placebo or brief resting periods followed by least three values. In each case the better two volumes differing by less than 5% for FVC and FEV_1, with the same requirements both before and after placebo. Table 5-3 gives the key published data of Sourk and Nugent[3] in1983 using 40 patients with obstructive airways disease with the following baseline values; age = 61 $\pm$ 11 years, FVC = 2.88 $\pm$ 0.92 L, FEV_1 1.63 $\pm$ 0.75 L and baseline FEV_1 percent of predicted = 60 $\pm$ 25%.

Sourk and Nugent[3] found (Table 5-3) that the mean differences between 3 pre-spirometric and 3 post-spirometric measures of FVC, FEV_1 and %FEV_1/FVC averaged about 1.0%. They calculated standard deviations of each set of measures as 5-8%. They then defined and calculated their upper confidence limits by using the mean plus variability of measurements between the pre-placebo and post-placebo administration and rest period. For example, the upper confidence limit for FVC = 1.27% + 6.7% $\times$ 2.02 = 14.9%. They interpreted these data and recommended that if a bronchodilator effect were to exceed normal variability, the value for a *single measure* of FVC would need to exceed the highest pre-bronchodilator measure by 14.9% and 340 mL; while the FEV_1 would need to exceed the highest pre-bronchodilator measure

Table 5-3	Changes in Spirometry After Placebo Inhalations[3]		
	Percent change after placebo		
Measure	Mean (%)	SD (%)	Upper confidence limits* (%)
FVC	1.27	6.7	14.9
FEV_1	0.97	5.6	12.3
FEV_1/FVC, %	0.57	8.0	16.7
	Absolute differences after placebo		
Measure	Mean difference	SD	Upper confidence limit*
FVC	25 mL	156 m	340 mL
FEV_1	10 mL	83 m	178 mL
FEV_1/FVC,%	0.40	4.03	8.55

*Ninety-five percent of the population is defined by the mean $\pm$ 2.02 standard deviations of the mean

by 12.3% and 178 mL, and the $\%FEV_1/FVC$ would need to exceed the highest pre-bronchodilator measure by 8.55% absolute or a relative 16.7% (The percent change required in $\%FEV_1/FVC$ seems especially suspicious as one very rarely if ever sees cooperative patients or normal individuals not in pain who change their $\%FEV_1/FVC$ by an average of 8% or 9% over a short time without cause).

Pellegrino et al.[4] measured the spirometric responses before and after placebo and brief rest in 26 patients with ages of 49 ± 16 years, FVC $86 \pm 18\%$ of predicted, and FEV_1 $63 \pm 19\%$ of predicted (Table 5-4). They used the same methods and statistical format as Sourk and Nugent (2.02 times SD plus mean difference is above 95% confidence limits).

Thus, again the mean pre-placebo and post-placebo measures of FVC and FEV_1 differed by less than 1%. However, they calculated that on average, for a *single measure* to exceed the population variability of their pre-placebo values, the FVC would, on average, need to increase 14% and 540 mL and the FEV_1, on average, 15% ($7\% \times 2.02 + 1\%$) and 250 ($120 \times 2 + 10$) mL.

Tweeddale et al.[5] measured the short-term variability in FEV_1 and FVC before and after a 20-minute rest period in 150 consecutive patients with obstructive ventilatory defects (Table 5-5). For each session they recorded three technically acceptable spirometric tracings and used the highest of these values in their calculations. They divided patients into three groups dependent on the absolute values of the best baseline FEV_1.

Absolute variability was calculated as post-prevalues and percent variability was calculated as (post-pre) $\times$ 100/mean of (post + pre). They reported that percent variability of FEV_1 and FVC both decreased significantly ($p < 0.001$ and $p = 0.001$)

Table 5-4	Spirometric Changes After Placebo Administration in 26 Patients[4]		
Measure	Mean (%)	SD (%)	Upper confidence limits*
FVC	−0.16	6.95	14%
FEV_1	1	7	15%
Measure	Mean difference	SD	Upper confidence limits*
FVC	−30 mL	260 mL	540 mL
FEV_1	+10 mL	120 mL	250 mL

*Ninety-five percent of the population is defined by the mean ± 2.02 standard deviations of the mean

Table 5-5	Natural Variability in FEV_1 and VC After a 20-minute Interval[5]		
	Group A	Group B	Group C
No. of patients	72	51	27
FEV_1 range, L	0.50–1.10	1.15–2.40	2.45–4.70
Absolute change, mL, mean	3	19	21
Absolute change, mL, SD	96	100	84
Percent change mean	−0.1	−1.6	−0.7
Percent change, SD	12.4	6.5	3.0
VC range, L	0.55–4.10	1.95–4.95	3.40–6.80
Absolute change, mL, mean	48	43	−46
Absolute change, mL, SD	211	189	181
Percent change, mean	2.6	1.3	−1.2
Percent change, SD	12.5	6.6	4.3

as absolute values of baseline FEV_1 and FVC increased. They then multiplied the average absolute variability of FEV_1 (~100 mL) and FVC (~200 mL) of all 150 patients times 1.645 ($p = 0.05$ for a one-tailed evaluation) and concluded that FEV_1 needed to change by 160 mL and FVC by 330 mL to significantly differ from baseline mean and variability.

Third, were the statistical analyses appropriate for deciding if three later samples are higher than three earlier samples? The author thinks the answer is negative. In each of these series, it seems that the analyses tried to translate for *a population*, how much a single new spirometric value needed to differ from the mean or higher values obtained from three prior samples in an individual. The analyses did not analyze for the difference between three pre-intervention samples and three postintervention samples. Notice also that to define statistical significance at about the 95% confidence limits, Tweeddale et al.[5] used 1.645, a one-tailed constant, whereas Sourk and Nugent[3] and Pellegrino et al.[4] used 2.02, a two-tailed constant to calculate of how much a *single* spirometric value should differ from the three pre-placebo mean or highest value.

ASSESSING DATA FROM THE HARBOR-UCLA LABORATORY

Hansen et al.[6] in 1993, reported the spirometric variability of 50 consecutive cooperative patients with FEV_1/FVC greater than 70% and mean baseline FEV_1 of 1.75 L. We measured FEV_1 at baseline, after aerosolized saline, or after aerosolized albuterol sulfate. In these patients, the absolute variability of FEV_1 for the 150 series of each set of five tests increased as mean FEV_1 increased while the percentage variability decreased (Table 5-6). The decline in percentage variability was similar to that of Tweeddale et al.[5]

In 2008, Hansen et al.[7] in other patients, reported data from the Harbor-UCLA laboratory regarding aerosolized bronchodilator responsiveness of over 300 consecutive patients, each with at least 2 of 3 forced expirations meeting ATS standards.[8] Some unpublished data from that second population is given in table 5-7. In each paired row, the table gives the mean values and variability of the lowest 10% of the patients versus the highest 10% of the patients, the difference between them by two-tailed *t*-tests, and the mean values and variability of the mid-80% of the patients. The purpose of this table is twofold. First (Parts A and B), in a population, variability is dependent on the absolute values of the FEV_1, FVC and their ratios. Second (Part C), the high variability of the FEV_1 values of a small portion of the population greatly affects the overall variability of the FEV_1, FVC and FEV_1/FVC of an entire population.

CRITIQUE OF ABOVE DATA

Absolute variability is measured by SD while percent variability is measured by %COV (100 × mean/SD). It is evident that:

- Absolute variability of FVC in a population is much greater than FEV_1 (Tables 5-3 to 5-5).
- As baseline FEV_1 increases in a population, the mean FVC, mean $\%FEV_1/FVC$ and SD of FEV_1 all increase, while the %COV of FEV_1, FVC and $\%FEV_1/FVC$ all markedly decrease (Figures 5-1 and 5-2 and Tables 5-6 and 5-7A).
- As $\%FEV_1/FVC$ decreases and obstruction increases in a population, the %COV of FEV_1, FVC and $\%FEV_1/FVC$ all increase, while the mean FEV_1 and FVC decrease (Table 5-7B). However, changes in $\%FEV_1/FVC$ should not be used as an indicator of acute bronchodilation, since major bronchodilation may occur with no change or a decline in FEV_1/FVC.

Table 5-6	Absolute and Percentage Variability of FEV_1 Measured Five Times in 50 Patients[6]		
FEV_1	Mean (L)	Mean SD (mL)	Mean COV (%)
	~0.50	32	6.4
	~1.00	40	4.0
	~1.50	48	3.2
	~2.00	56	2.8
	~2.50	64	2.6
	~3.00	72	2.4
	~3.50	80	2.3
Population mean	1.75 L	51	3.0

- As the % COV of FEV_1 increases (Table 5-7C), the percent variability of all measures increase.
- The raw data of SD and %COV values shown in figures 5-1 and 5-2 and the data in table 5-7 show that the great majority (approximately 90%) of individual values are much less than the mean variability reported in other series in tables 5-3 to 5-5. After noting the red COV values in all parts of table 5-7, it is clear that 90% of all patients have %COV which are less than 3.0%. These values times 1.645 are less than 5.0%. This means that in 90% of patients we studied, a change of over 5% is likely to be statistically significant using a one-tailed t-test. Thus, it appears that a minority of individuals in the population studied account for the high absolute and percent variability found in other series. The values displayed in the table 5-7 series, which give the mean variabilities of the lower and higher 10% of all 317 individuals measured and the values in table 5-7 strongly suggest that the calculated population values of the three series may be inappropriate to use when interpreting data from individual patients.
- In fact, the required changes for a positive response reported by these three series generally exceeds by wide margins; the variability found in the most variable 10% of patients in the Harbor-UCLA series.
- Furthermore, if one used the calculated numbers of tables 5-3 to 5-5, it is reasonable to recommend that the requirements for bronchodilation for FEV_1 using old population values should be volume *or* percentage based rather than volume *and* percentage based, and that the volumes for FEV_1 should be lower than those for FVC, as the latter is exhalation time dependent. In the past, FEV_3 and FEV_6 values were not usually tabulated and considered, but they have the advantage with FEV_1 of not being dependent on the duration of expiration, as are FVC values.

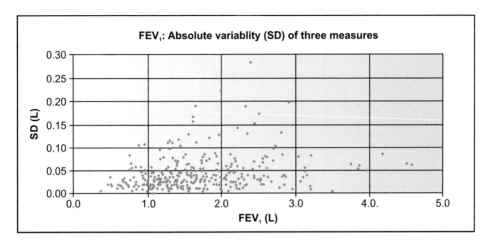

Figure 5-1 Variability of SD of FEV$_1$ values in 317 patients prior to receiving aerosolized salbutamol. As values of FEV$_1$ increased, absolute variability as measured by SD generally increased.

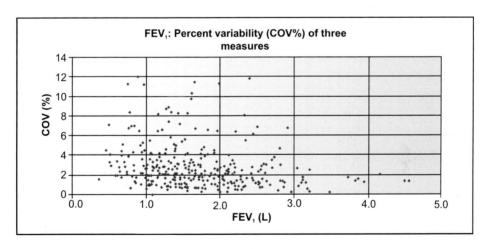

Figure 5-2 Percent variability of FEV$_1$ values in 317 patients prior to receiving aerosolized salbutamol. As values of FEV$_1$ increased, percentage variability as measured by percent coefficient of variation (COV) generally decreased.

Wisely, the committees reviewing these data claimed only clinical significance and carefully did not claim "statistical significance" for their recommendations. They may well have considered that despite the statistical derived requirements of up to 540 mL (Table 5-4), these values were unrealistic. It is surprising that they

Table 5-7 Pre-Bronchodilator Spirometric Values and Variability in 317 Consecutive Harbor-UCLA Patients*

	Age	FVC (mL)			FEV$_1$ (mL)			%FEV$_1$/FVC		
	Mean	Mean	SD	COV	Mean	SD	COV	Mean	SD	COV
A. Sorted by FEV$_1$										
Lo 0.1	62	1,360	64	4.80%	680	28	3.98%	53.1%	2.08%	3.92%
Mid 0.8	57	2,410	69	2.88%	1,630	50	2.56%	66.6%	1.74%	2.70%
Hi 0.1	44	4,260	61	1.46%	3,190	57	1.84%	75.1%	1.39%	1.88%
p =	0.00001	0.00001	NS	0.00001	0.00001	0.0004	0.0003	0.00001	NS	0.00001
B. Sorted by %FEV$_1$/FVC										
Lo 0.1	61	2,420	110	4.62%	960	38	3.85%	40.4	1.81%	4.48%
Mid 0.8	57	2330	63	2.75%	1710	45	2.82%	67.4%	1.77%	2.65%
Hi 0.1	51	2,690	64	2.59%	2,230	50	2.39%	81.6	1.49%	1.82%
p =	0.0006	NS	0.002	0.0007	0.00001	NS	0.002	0.00001	NS	0.00001
C. Sorted by variability of FEV$_1$										
Lo 0.1	55	2,790	50	1.89%	1,970	10	0.54%	70.3	1.28%	1.88%
Mid 0.8	57	2,520	64	2.75%	1,680	39	2.45%	66.3%	1.59%	2.52%
Hi 0.1	57	2,420	116	5.22%	1,480	122	8.29%	61.3	3.30%	5.30%
p =	NS	NS	0.00001	0.00001	0.03	0.00001	0.00001	0.0008	0.00001	0.00001

*The Lo (Low) 0.1, Mid (Medium) 0.8, and Hi (High) 0.1 rows display the mean values of their measures, their SD's and their Coefficient of Variation (COV) of the lowest and highest 10% of the 317 patients. The Mid 0.8 rows display the same information for the majority (80%) of the remaining population. The p-values for the lower versus higher ten percents of the patient are calculated from two-tailed unpaired t-tests. Those emboldened have the most important p-values. The weighted average of the two red values in each combination indicates the variability of the less variable 90% of each group of 317. In every grouping, the average COV for the better 90% of the population is below 2.8%

selected 200 mL as a requirement for both FEV_1 and FVC and more surprising that they required both volume *and* percentage changes. As you will note in specific patients later by: (1) requiring a volume change of 200 mL to conclude that there is a positive bronchodilator effect penalizes severely ill patients, and (2) requiring a volume change of 12% to conclude there is a positive bronchodilator effect penalizes individuals with large baseline volumes.

PRACTICAL AND LEGITIMATE STATISTICAL ANALYSES AND RECOMMENDATIONS

Finally these published population differences between pre- and post-placebo spirometric variables are of limited relevance in evaluating bronchodilator responsiveness in individual patients. As is almost self-evident, individuals, especially those with obstructive airway disease, differ markedly in their baseline variability. Rather than relying on older, easily misinterpreted, and complicated population-based statistics, it makes much more sense to rely on a valid statistical analysis of each individual patient, especially since those data are readily available right in the laboratory. Such an analysis is simple, especially since the performance of three satisfactory pre-tests and three satisfactory post-tests already is standard practice in pulmonary laboratories.

Reporting the results of that statistical analysis to the referring physician is the optimal way to transmit useful information. This can be done by unpaired one- or two-tailed *t*-testing, or by rank order testing which can be done quickly without a calculator (For example, see the tables in section: Analyzing Individual Patient Data). In my opinion, the laboratory physician should not recommend to the referring physician if a drug should or should not be used. Rather, the laboratory physician should report the consistency or inconsistency of the response, and the degree of the response, if any, to a given aerosolized drug or combination of aerosolized drugs. The clinician, considering all aspects of the patient's health or illness and the potential positive and/or negative effects of using aerosolized drugs, must decide whether or not to use specific drugs.

Rank order testing is simple but requires six values to reach statistical significance at the $p = 0.05$ level: three pre-BD and three post-BD.[9] If the three individual FEV_1 post-BD are all larger than all three of the FEV_1 pre-BD values, then that combination gives a p-value for FEV_1 of exactly 0.05 (Seven or more values are needed to reach a p-value < 0.05).[9] This can be interpreted as a consistent and statistically significant change. If there is any tie between pre- and post-BD values, or if any pre-BD value exceeds any post-BD value, then $p > 0.05$ and this should be interpreted as an inconsistent or insignificant change after BD. I also look at the changes in FEV_3 and

Table 5-8	Changes from Pre- to Post-Bronchodilator Therapy in Four Theoretical Cases			
Patient	Pre-BD (mL)	Post-BD (mL)	Absolute volume change (mL)	Percentage volume change
A	600	700	100	17
B	3000	3100	100	3
C	600	800	200	33
D	3000	4000	1000	33

BD, bronchodilator

FVC or FEV_6 if that is recorded. Ideally, and well over 19/20 of the time, the changes in FEV_3 and FEV_6 parallel those of FEV_1 and are of the same statistical significance. The FVC values are somewhat different, as the values in each forced exhalation are dependent on the duration of the FVC. If the FEV_1 does not change post-BD and the FVC increases, that is usually due to longer exhalations rather than true bronchodilation. Besides consistency, the degree of change is relevant.

Regardless of the volume change it seems reasonable to interpret increases in FEV_1 of less than 3% as trivial, 3–6% as minimal, 6–12% as mild, 12–24% as moderate and > 24% as marked, but these percentages are arbitrary. It also seems reasonable, from the patient's viewpoint, to consider percentage change more important than volume change. If we consider four theoretical cases, I think it likely that patients A, C, and D showed significant improvement from an aerosolized bronchodilator but that patient B did not, unless that he was a competitive athlete (Table 5-8).

ANALYZING DATA FROM A SINGLE POPULATION: COMPARING TWO METHODS

In order to compare ATS/ERS guidelines with individual patient statistical analyses, we retrospectively analyzed data from consecutive patients in a calendar year who received nebulized albuterol in our clinical laboratory.[7] To be included, each had to have 2 or 3 of 3 pre-BD studies plus 2 or 3 of 3 post-BD studies meeting ATS quality standards.[8] If the patient increased their best post-BD FEV_1 or FVC by both 200 mL and 12%, that patient was considered to be ATS/ERS guideline positive (A⁺), if not, ATS/ERS guideline negative (A⁻).

One-Tailed t-Tests

Alternatively, one can use unpaired one-tailed t-tests to compare the pre- and post-BD studies. If a patient increased their FEV_1 plus FEV_3 or FVC by $p > 0.05$, that patient was considered to be Harbor guideline positive (H⁺), if not, Harbor guideline negative (H⁻). The 313 patients fit into the following groups: 135 or 43% were A⁻ and H⁻ (true negative), 86 or 27% were A⁺ and H⁺ (true positive), 89 or 28% were A⁻H⁺ (false negative) and 3 or 1% were A⁺H⁻ (false positive). Thus, there were rare false positives and slightly more A⁻H⁺ than A⁺H⁺, meaning that statistically significant bronchodilation was observed in 89 patients who did not meet the ATS/ERS guideline criteria for bronchodilation (Table 5-9).

Figure 5-3 displays the results according to the baseline FEV₁ volume. The few patients considered positive by ATS/ERS guidelines and negative by Harbor

Table 5-9	Analysis of Responses of 313 Patients to Aerosolized Bronchodilator	
Results	ATS/ERS positive	ATS/ERS negative
Harbor positive	True positive 86 (27%)	False negative 89 (28%)
Harbor negative	False positive 3 (1%)	True negative 135 (43%)

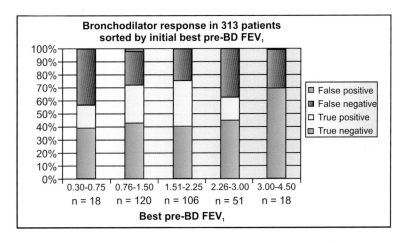

Figure 5-3 Bronchodilator response in 313 patients receiving aerosolized albuterol sorted by severity of baseline FEV₁ (0.3–4.5 L) into five groups (columns) of 18, 120, 106, 51, and 18 patients. In green are patients who did not meet ATS/ERS guidelines nor Harbor guidelines for bronchodilation (A⁻, H⁻, true negatives); in yellow are those who met both ATS/ERS and Harbor guidelines (A⁺, H⁺, true positives); in pink are those who did not meet ATS/ERS guidelines but did meet Harbor guidelines (A⁻, H⁺, false negatives) and in blue are those who met ATS/ERS guidelines but did not meet Harbor guidelines (A⁺, H⁻, false positives).[7]

guidelines (A$^+$H$^-$) had > 200 mL increases in FVC post-BD, attributable to longer post-BD exhalations, but not in FEV$_1$. The false negatives (A$^-$H$^+$) predominated in those with very low FEV$_1$ < 0.75 L because they did not meet the 200 mL criterion, or those with large FEV$_1$ > 2.25 L, because they did not meet the 12% criterion. No patient with a baseline FEV$_1$ of 3.00 L or more met the ATS/ERS criteria. Twenty-four percent of the A$^-$H$^+$ patients did not meet the ATS/ERS 200 mL criterion but met percentage change criterion; 16% met the 12% criterion but not the volume criterion. Thus, if the ATS/ERS criteria were changed from "AND to OR", 40% of the patients who were false negatives by ATS/ERS guidelines would have been accepted as positive bronchodilation responses.

Rank Order Testing

It is useful to compare rank order testing with one-tailed t-testing in evaluating tree pre-BD and three post-BD FEV$_1$, FEV$_3$, FEV$_6$ or FVC volumes. t-testing requires more complex calculations than simple rank order testing, which is only feasible if there are a total of three pre-BD and three post-BD tests. If all three post-BD values are higher than all three pre-BD values, without any ties, the $p = 0.05$ by rank order

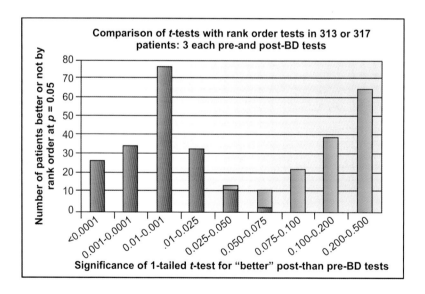

Figure 5-4 Comparison of two-tailed t-test values with rank order values in 313 patients for changes in FEV$_1$ values from three pre- to three post-aerosolized albuterol (BD). P-values ranged from < 0.0001 to 0.500. Rank order values could only be $p = 0.05$ (considered significant) or $p > 0.05$ (considered insignificant). Note concordance in 99% of patients.[7]

testing. Figure 5-4 shows the excellent matching between a $p < 0.05$ to $p < 0.0001$ on t-tests and $p = 0.05$ on rank order tests and also the excellent matching of $p > 0.5$ to $p = 0.50$ on t-tests and $p > 0.05$ on rank order tests. There were dissimilar findings in only three comparisons, when t-test values were between 0.028 and 0.075. Most of the H^+ patients had p-values on unpaired one-tailed t-tests of $p < 0.01$ while by rank order testing p-values cannot be lower than $p = 0.05$ when only six values are available. Thus rank-order statistics, which are easy to perform, offer a quick way to decide whether or not the pre-BD and post-BD values are significantly different.

ANALYZING INDIVIDUAL PATIENT DATA

Following are several examples (Tables 5-10 to 5-21) of how actual patient data from the pulmonary laboratory can be interpreted by the laboratory physician to the physician caring for the patient. The first table of each pair includes an

Table 5-10	Analyzing Data from Patient Number 1 (61-year-old Latin Woman, 149 cm Tall)					
Three trials	FEV_1 (L)		FEV_3 (L)		FVC (L)	
	Pre-BD	Post-BD	Pre-BD	Post-BD	Pre-BD	Post-BD
Max	0.62	0.76			1.06	1.256
Max, abs Δ	0.14		0.18		0.19	
Max % Δ	22.6%		21.4%		17.9%	

ATS/ERS guideline interpretation: Severe obstructive lung disease. Increases in FEV_1 and FVC are less than 200 mL after aerosolized bronchodilator. Therefore, there is no significant change. This does not preclude use of bronchodilator therapy.

Table 5-11	More Complete Data from Patient Number 1 (61-year-old Latin Woman, 149 cm Tall)					
Trials	FEV_1 (L)		FEV_3 (L)		FVC (L)	
	Pre-BD	Post-BD	Pre-BD	Post-BD	Pre-BD	Post-BD
1	0.58	0.73	0.79	0.98	0.87	1.16
2	0.61	0.76	0.82	1.02	1.03	1.25
3	0.62	0.76	0.84	1.01	1.06	1.21
Max	0.62	0.76	0.84	1.02	10.6	1.25
Max, abs Δ	0.14		0.18		0.19	
Max % Δ	22.6%		21.4%		17.9%	
t-test $p =$	0.0004		0.0003		0.013	
Rank order $p =$	0.05		0.05		0.05	

Harbor interpretation: Severe obstructive lung disease. There are consistent, moderate, and statistically significant improvements in FEV_1, FEV_3, and FVC after aerosolized bronchodilator.

Table 5-12	Analyzing Data from Patient Number 2 (67-year-old White Woman, 169 cm Tall)					

TLC Act/Pred = 4.40/4.75				**DLCO Act/Pred = 8.0/22.7**		
Three trials	FEV_1 (L)		FEV_3 (L)		FVC (L)	
	Pre-BD	Post-BD	Pre-BD	Post-BD	Pre-BD	Post-BD
Max	0.85	0.96	1.16	1.24	1.31	1.43
Max, abs Δ	0.11		0.06		0.12	
Max % Δ	12.9%		6.9%		9.2%	

ATS/ERS guideline interpretation: Severe obstructive lung disease with severe loss of pulmonary capillary vasculature. Increases in FEV_1 and FVC are less than 200 mL after aerosolized bronchodilator. Therefore, there is no significant change. This does not preclude use of bronchodilator therapy.

Table 5-13	More Complete Data from Patient Number 2 (67-year-old White Woman, 169 cm Tall)					

TLC Act/Pred = 4.40/4.75				**DLCO Act/Pred = 8.0/22.7**		
Trials	FEV_1 (L)		FEV_3 (L)		FVC (L)	
	Pre-BD	Post-BD	Pre-BD	Post-BD	Pre-BD	Post-BD
1	0.84	0.92	1.16	1.24	1.31	1.43
2	0.81	0.96	1.11	1.23	1.19	1.38
3	0.85	0.90	1.16	1.22	1.22	1.42
Max	0.85	0.96	1.16	1.24	1.31	1.43
Max, abs Δ	0.11		0.08		0.12	
Max % Δ	12.9%		6.9%		9.2%	
t-test $p =$	0.006		0.004		0.006	
Rank order $p =$	0.05		0.05		0.05	

Harbor interpretation: Severe obstructive lung disease with severe loss of pulmonary capillary vasculature. There are consistent, mild, and statistically significant improvements in FEV_1, FEV_3 and FVC after aerosolized bronchodilator.

Table 5-14	Analyzing Data from Patient Number 3 (54-year-old White Man, 198 cm Tall)					

				DLCO Act/Pred = 43.6/36.0		
Three trials	FEV_1 (L)		FEV_3 (L)		FVC (L)	
	Pre-BD	Post-BD	Pre-BD	Post-BD	Pre-BD	Post-BD
Max	3.86	4.28	5.03	5.36	5.72	6.06
Max, abs Δ	0.42		0.33		0.34	
Max % Δ	10.9%		6.6%		5.6%	

ATS/ERS guideline interpretation: Mild obstructive lung disease with mildly increased DLCO. Absolute increases in FEV_1 and FVC are less than 12% after aerosolized bronchodilator. Therefore, there is no significant change. This does not preclude use of bronchodilator therapy.

Table 5-15	More Complete Data from Patient Number 3 (54-year-old White Man, 198 cm Tall)					
					DLCO Act/Pred = 43.6/36.0	
Trials	FEV$_1$ (L)		FEV$_3$ (L)		FVC (L)	
	Pre-BD	Post-BD	Pre-BD	Post-BD	Pre-BD	Post-BD
1	3.86	4.26	5.03	5.34	5.72	5.92
2	3.84	4.28	5.02	5.36	5.71	6.06
3	3.76	4.23	4.95	5.28	5.66	6.04
Max	3.86	4.28	5.03	5.36	5.72	6.06
Max, abs Δ	0.42		0.33		0.34	
Max % Δ	10.9%		8.6%		5.6%	
t-test p =	0.001		0.0004		0.016	
Rank order p =	0.05		0.05		0.05	

Harbor interpretation: Mild obstructive lung disease with mild, consistent, and statistically significant improvement in FEV$_1$, FEV$_3$ and FVC after aerosolized bronchodilator. The DLCO is mildly elevated. The findings are consistent with asthma.

Table 5-16	Analyzing Data from Patient Number 4 (65-year-old Black Woman, 157 cm Tall)					
TLC Act/Pred = 3.86/3.95			**DLCO Act/Pred = 2.0/20.5**			
Three trials	FEV$_1$ (L)		FEV$_3$ (L)		FVC (L)	
	Pre-BD	Post-BD	Pre-BD	Post-BD	Pre-BD	Post-BD
Max	1.16	1.32	1.68	1.89	2.16	2.26
Max, abs Δ	0.16		0.21		0.12	
Max % Δ	13.8%		12.5%		5.6%	

ATS/ERS guideline interpretation: Severe obstructive lung disease with very severe loss of pulmonary capillary vasculature. Absolute increases in FEV$_1$ and FVC are less than 0.2 L after aerosolized bronchodilator. Therefore, there is no significant change. This does not preclude use of bronchodilator therapy.

Table 5-17	More Complete Data from Patient Number 4 (65-year-old Black Woman, 157 cm Tall)					
TLC Act/Pred = 3.86/3.95				**DLCO Act/Pred = 2.0/20.5**		
Trials	FEV_1 (L)		FEV_3 (L)		FVC (L)	
	Pre-BD	Post-BD	Pre-BD	Post-BD	Pre-BD	Post-BD
1	1.15	1.25	1.67	1.86	2.13	2.24
2	1.12	1.25	1.61	1.85	2.13	2.28
3	1.16	1.32	1.68	1.89	2.16	2.27
Max	1.16	1.32	1.68	1.89	2.16	2.28
Max, abs Δ	0.16		0.21		0.12	
Max % Δ	13.8%		12.6%		5.6%	
t-test p =	0.001		0.0005		0.001	
Rank order p =	0.05		0.05		0.05	

Harbor interpretation: Severe obstructive lung disease with very severe loss of pulmonary capillary vasculature. There are consistent, moderate and statistically significant improvements in FEV_1 and FEV_3 after aerosolized bronchodilator.

Table 5-18	Analyzing Data from Patient Number 5 (70-year-old Black Man, 163 cm Tall)					
TLC Act/Pred = 7.58/5.09				**DLCO Act/Pred = 4.3/21.4**		
Three trials	FEV_1 (L)		FEV_3 (L)		FVC (L)	
	Pre-BD	Post-BD	Pre-BD	Post-BD	Pre-BD	Post-BD
Max	0.81	0.91	1.33	1.46	2.46	2.55
Max, abs Δ	0.10		0.13		0.09	
Max % Δ	12.4%		9.8%		3.7%	

ATS/ERS guideline interpretation: Severe obstructive disease with hyperinflation and severe loss of pulmonary capillary vasculature. Absolute increases in FEV_1 and FVC are less than 0.2 L after aerosolized bronchodilator. Therefore, there is no significant change. This does not preclude use of bronchodilator therapy.

Table 5-19	More Complete Data from Patient Number 5 (70-year-old Black Man, 163 cm Tall)					
TLC Act/Pred = 7.58/5.09				**DLCO Act/Pred = 4.3/21.4**		
Trials	FEV$_1$ (L)		FEV$_3$ (L)		FVC (L)	
	Pre-BD	Post-BD	Pre-BD	Post-BD	Pre-BD	Post-BD
1	0.71	0.90	1.18	1.46	2.22	2.46
2	0.81	0.89	1.33	1.44	2.46	2.65
3	0.74	0.91	1.23	1.46	2.39	2.62
Max	0.81	0.91	1.33	1.46	2.46	2.65
Max, abs Δ	0.10		0.13		0.11	
Max % Δ	12.4%		9.8%		6.4%	
t-test p =	0.001		0.005		0.014	
Rank order p =	0.05		0.05		> 0.05	

Harbor interpretation: Severe obstructive lung disease with hyperinflation and severe loss of pulmonary capillary vasculature. There are consistent, mild to moderate, and statistically significant improvements in FEV$_1$ and FEV$_3$ after aerosolized bronchodilator.

Table 5-20	Analyzing Data from Patient Number 6 (76-year-old Asian Woman, 143 cm Tall)					
TLC Act/Pred = 4.59/3.49				**DLCO Act/Pred = 13.4/15.8**		
Three trials	FEV$_1$ (L)		FEV$_3$ (L)		FVC (L)	
	Pre-BD	Post-BD	Pre-BD	Post-BD	Pre-BD	Post-BD
Max	0.75	0.82	1.21	1.29	1.71	1.82
Max, abs Δ	0.07		0.08		0.11	
Max % Δ	9.3%		6.6%		6.4%	

ATS/ERS guideline interpretation: Severe obstructive disease. Absolute increases in FEV$_1$ and FVC are less than 0.2 L after aerosolized bronchodilator. Therefore, there is no significant change. This does not preclude use of bronchodilator therapy.

interpretation based on ATS/ERS guidelines. The second table of each pair includes the data available to the laboratory physician and an interpretation using guidelines suggested in this chapter. Please study these to see the different messages that might be received by the referring physician. The alternate messages received by the referring physician depend on whether the laboratory physician (1) uses the ATS/ERS guidelines or (2) reviews the actual data and analyses them statistically. If you were the referring physician, which would you prefer?

Table 5-21	More Complete Data from Patient Number 6 (76-year-old Asian Woman, 143 cm Tall)					
TLC Act/Pred = 4.59/3.49				DLCO Act/Pred = 13.4/15.8		
Trials	FEV_1 (L)		FEV_3 (L)		FVC (L)	
	Pre-BD	Post-BD	Pre-BD	Post-BD	Pre-BD	Post-BD
1	0.75	0.77	1.21	1.24	1.58	1.75
2	0.73	0.82	1.20	1.29	1.65	1.82
3	0.72	0.81	1.17	1.26	1.71	1.82
Max	0.75	0.82	1.21	1.29	1.71	1.82
Max, abs Δ	0.07		0.08		0.11	
Max % Δ	9.3%		6.6%		6.4%	
t-test p =	0.01		0.01		0.014	
Rank order p =	0.05		0.05		0.05	

Harbor interpretation: Severe obstructive lung disease with hyperinflation and severe loss of pulmonary capillary vasculature. There are consistent, mild and statistically significant improvements in FEV_1, FEV_3, and FVC after aerosolized bronchodilator.

BRONCHIAL PROVOCATION TESTING

General

Bronchial provocation testing is useful for inducing evidence of hyperresponsive airways in patients with normal spirometry but clinically suspected of having asthma. After preliminary baseline measurement of FEV_1, increasing dosages of methacholine or adenosine triphosphate or mannitol or an equivalent irritant aerosolized agent are introduced into the airway of the patient alternating with repeated forced exhalations. If reductions in airflow occur at low dosages, that finding is usually interpreted as being supportive of the diagnosis of reactive airways disease or asthma. If reductions in airflow do not occur at high dosages, this finding is usually interpreted as indicating the absence of reactive airways or asthma. Occasionally, in suspected occupationally induced asthma, suspected specific allergens rather than methacholine are introduced to test airway responsiveness to them.

Procedure

For several to 48 hours before testing inhaled and oral agents which could cause bronchodilation (including corticosteroids, beta agonists, cromolyn, and antihistamines) are withheld. The challenging agent is prepared in multiple dilutions for aerosol administration and is delivered in increasing dosages for five inhalations,

3 minutes rest, two forced spirometric exhalations, evaluation of the expiratory values, and repetition at a higher dilution if there is no important reduction in FEV_1. Each of the five inhalations of the aerosolized drug uses a full vital capacity maneuver with breath-holding at TLC for 2-5 seconds. If the reduction in FEV_1 is less than 20% at 3-6 minutes after each set of 5 inhalations, the next higher dosage of methacholine (or other drug) is used for five inhalations as before. Successive dilutions of methacholime in mg/mL might be: 0.000 (the diluent without methacholine), 0.075, 0.15, 0.3, 0.6, 1.2, 2.5, 5, 10 and 25 mg/mL.

Higher dosages of methacholine should not be administered if the FEV_1 falls 20% or more below baseline. If the patient experiences any distress, albuterol or other beta agonist should be administered by aerosol and the patient followed in the laboratory until the FEV_1 has returned to baseline.

Interpretation

Normal individuals usually have little or no reduction in FEV_1 even with dosages of 25 mg/mL of methacholine. Asthmatics usually have a reduction of FEV_1 of 20% (often identified as provocative concentration or PC20) or more well before this concentration of methacholine. Individuals with chronic bronchitis may also manifest moderate responsiveness. There is unlikely to be more useful information obtained by repeated measurements of $FEF_{25-75\%}$ or total lung capacity.

Other Resources

More detailed information can be found in guideline publications of the European Thoracic Society[10] and American Thoracic Society.[11]

EXERCISE-INDUCED ASTHMA

General

Exercise-induced asthma (EIA) is relatively common in younger individuals, especially athletes. Several Olympic Gold-medal-winning swimmers have had EIA. In such individuals, symptoms of shortness of breath, with or without wheezing, tend to occur with intense exercise or immediately thereafter. High humidity and warm air tend to inhibit EIA, explaining why swimming is a preferred sport for those who have EIA. The EIA is most likely to be induced with outdoor exercise, where dust and pollens are most prevalent, or in extremely cold climates, where the humidity is very low even if there is snow in the air. It is more difficult to develop EIA in the laboratory environment, especially when using cycle rather than treadmill exercise.

Procedure

For several to 24 hours before testing inhaled and oral agents which could cause bronchodilation (including corticosteroids, beta agonists, cromolyn and antihistamines) are withheld. Spirometric measurements of FEV_1 should be made immediately before and again immediately and for several minutes after intense outdoor exercise, e.g., running on a track or in a field. Measurement of heart rate by some method is desirable. In the laboratory, the patient suspected of having asthma should have measurements of FEV_1, have ECG recordings, and then exercise vigorously for 4–6 minutes until exhaustion or near exhaustion or the development of wheezing or significant shortness of breath. During the exercise period, it is appropriate to start with lower intensity exercise and then rapidly increase it to the patient's tolerance. A mouthpiece or mask can be utilized to collect metabolic data (e.g., ventilation, oxygen uptake, carbon dioxide output, etc.), but it is preferable for the subject to breath in cold or non-humidified room air without a mouthpiece or mask. If metabolic measurements are made, the mask or mouthpiece should be removed as soon as the patient stops exercise so that the first forced expiratory maneuver can be recorded. It is reasonable to perform and measure forced expiratory maneuvers at 1, 3, 5, and 10 minutes. The forced expiratory maneuvers need not last longer than 3 seconds; it is not necessary to measure FVC. If the decline in FEV_1 is marked or the patient is distressed, an inhaled beta-agonist can be administered to relieve the bronchospasm.

Interpretation

If the patient has EIA, the FEV_1 usually declines by 15% or more during the recovery period after the intense exercise. Entirely normal individuals tend to have little or no decline in FEV_1 and sometimes a minimal improvement in FEV_1 during the post-exercise period.

CONCLUSION

For bronchodilator testing it is recommended that those physicians who have access to the data for each forced expiration, review the FEV_1, FEV_3 and FEV_6 for the three best before-BD and three best after-BD tests. In assessing bronchodilation, it is also reasonable to consider the FVC, although the FVC can change as a result of the duration of exhalation. If you refer patients to laboratories who do not use the data of all forced exhalations in their interpretations or do not offer you access to these data, it is suggested that you might alert them regarding the usefulness of this information to you, the referring physician.

REFERENCES

1. American Thoracic Society. Lung function testing: selection of reference values and interpretative strategies. *Am Rev Respir Dis*. 1991;144:1202-18.

2. Pelligrino R, Viegi G, Brusasco V, et al. Interpretative strategies for lung function tests. *Eur Respir J*. 2005;26:948-68.

3. Sourk RL, Nugent KM. Bronchodilator testing: confidence intervals derived from placebo inhalations. *Am Rev Respir Dis*. 1983;128:153-7.

4. Pelligrino R, Rodarte JR, Brusasco V. Assessing the reversibility of airway obstruction. *Chest*. 1998;114:1607-12.

5. Tweeddale PM, Alexander F, McHardy GJR. Short term variability in FEV_1 and bronchodilator responsiveness in patients with obstructive ventilatory defects. *Thorax*. 1987;42:487-90.

6. Hansen JE, Casaburi R, Goldberg AS. A statistical approach for assessment of bronchodilator responsiveness in pulmonary function testing. *Chest*. 1993;104:1119-28.

7. Hansen JE, Sun XG, Adame D, et al. Argument for changing criteria for bronchodilator responsiveness. *Respir Med*. 2008;102:1777-83.

8. American Thoracic Society. Standardization of spirometry: 1994 update. *Am J Respir Crit Care Med*. 1995;152:1107-36.

9. Dixon WJ, Massey FJ. Introduction to Statistical Analysis, 3rd edition. New York: McGraw Hill; 1969.

10. Sterk PJ, Fabbri RM, Quanjer PH, et al. Airway responsiveness. Standard challenge testing with pharmacological, physical, and sensitizing stimuli in adults. Report Working Party Standardization of Lung Function Tests, European Community for Steel and Coal.Official Statement of the European Respiratory Society. *Eur Respir J Suppl*. 1993;16:53-83.

11. Crapo RO, Casaburi R, Coates AL, et al. Guidelines for methacholine and exercise challenge testing – 1999. *Am J Respir Crit Care Med*. 2000;161:309-29.

6 Lung Volume Measurement

INTRODUCTION

Some lung volumes within the VC are measured with spirometry alone. As previously noted (Chapter 2), combinations of volumes are identified as capacities, so that VT + IRV = IC; IC + ERV = VC, and ERV + RV = FRC. The RV and TLC are rarely directly measured in the laboratory. Rather FRC is directly measured and RV and TLC are calculated as follows. RV = FRC – ERV and TLC = IC + FRC. In contrast to the VC or FVC, which are always the maximal values validly measured: all other lung volumes and capacities are reported as the averages of the validly measured volumes.

Sometimes incorrectly, a technician or physician measures the largest rather than average IC which they subtract from VC to determine the ERV. Correctly, the sum of the average IC and average ERV values together must equal the VC. Similarly, the final acceptable FRC measurement values must be the average of whatever valid measurements are made, not the largest recorded values. The RV is the average FRC minus the average ERV; the TLC is the average FRC plus the average IC. Although there are several publications which give predicting equations for ERV determined from FRC – RV equations, it is far more direct and valid to measure ERV and IC from spirometry tracings where VT and VC are recorded.

PLETHYSMOGRAPHY: THEORY AND PRACTICE

Theory of Measurement

Body plethysmography is an ingenious method of measuring FRC developed by DuBois and Comroe[1] in the 1940s and 1950s using a modified airtight Navy steel chamber as the "body box". DuBois[2] used the concept that, in a closed inflexible "box" with two compartments, the pressure times volume in one compartment was competitive with and reflected the pressure times volume in the other compartment, i.e., the lung. If a subject quietly seated within a box of approximately 600 L made panting maneuvers against a closed shutter, thereby changing the pressures and volumes within the thorax, the pressures and volumes within the box would also change synchronously. The pressures could then be recorded against each other on an X-Y recorder. There were three additional factors: (1) Within the box, body heat continuously warmed the air in the box so that the box had to be vented frequently so that the pressure of the gases were relatively stable for the second or two when the panting maneuvers were recorded. (2) The measurements of box pressure change required extremely sensitive pressure transducers since the pressure changes around the subject in the 600 L box were less than 1/100th of the pressure changes within the thorax during the panting maneuvers. (3) The volume of the air in the box was reduced by the volume of the patient or subject in the box. Since body density is close to 1.07 L/kg, the reduction in box volume could be estimated by considering the body weight of the patient as below:

$$PV = \text{Constant with stable temperature}$$
$$P_1 \times V_1 = (P_1 + \Delta P) \times (V_1 + \Delta V)$$

Consider $P_1 = P_{Box}$ and $V_1 = V_{TG}$ = Trapped gas volume FRC, if shutter closed properly.

Then, $$P_{Box} \times V_{TG} = P_{Box} \times V_{TG} + \Delta P \times V_{TG} + P_{Box} \times \Delta V + \Delta V \times \Delta P$$

Then, $$P_{Box} \times V_{TG} - P_{Box} \times V_{TG} = \Delta P \times V_{TG} + P_{Box} \times \Delta V + \Delta V \times \Delta P$$

Then, $$0 = \Delta P \times V_{TG} + P_{Box} \times \Delta V + \Delta V \times \Delta P$$

Then, ignoring $\Delta V \times \Delta P$,

$$V_{TG} = - P_{Box} \times \Delta V / \Delta P$$

Making the Measurement

The technician making measurements asks the subject to hold his/her cheeks so that they do not inflate and deflate markedly during the panting and encourages the subject to "pant" at a rate between 60 and 90 per minute even though, with the panting, no air escapes from the patient. The thoracic pressure is usually recorded on the Y-axis while the box pressure is recorded on the X-axis. The scales are adjusted so that if the recorded slope is steep, the thoracic gas volume is low; if the slope is shallow, the thoracic gas volume is high. In order to measure FRC directly, the technician must close the shutter at the end of a quiet expiratory breath. Currently, the software which records breathing volumes corrects for the differences between the "trapped gas volume (V_{TG})" and the volume of the patient's actual FRC. Nowadays, attractive, large-windowed "boxes" are available. Thus, several measurements of FRC can be measured and averaged into a final value. The RV is calculated from FRC – average ERV. The TLC is calculated from FRC plus average IC. Figure 6-1 shows an example of tracings the V_{TG} which in this instance, because the shutter was closed at end expiration, is equivalent to the subjects FRC.

Calculations

The empty body "box" is calibrated using a reciprocating pump syringe with a volume change of perhaps 30 mL of air which creates pressure changes within the

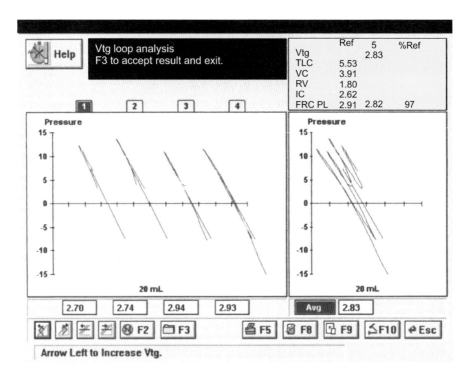

Figure 6-1 Plethysmographic measurement of FRC on an X-Y recorder screen with changes in mouth (alveolar) pressure plotted on the Y-axis and changes in box pressure plotted on the X-axis during panting maneuvers against a closed shutter. On the left, four separate tracings are shown with reasonably similar findings of V_{TG} of 2.70, 2.74, 2.94 and 2.93 L, with an average, on the right of 2.83 L. Since the shutter before panting was closed at the end of normal tidal breathing, the FRC is calculated as 2.82 L.

closed box measured by the sensitive pressure transducer. The pressure changes are somewhat similar to those expected when the patient pants against a closed shutter. As noted before, the volume of air in the empty "box" is reduced when a subject is seated in the box by a volume in liters times 1.07, since weight in kilograms times 1.07 approximates the subject's body volume. The pressure changes in the reduced box volume (ΔP_{BOX}) and mouth behind the closed shutter (ΔP_{mouth}) are used in calculations of the V_{TG} behind the shutter when the patient pants.

When box pressure has been stabilized by venting,[3] if Box volume = 530 L; subject's weight = 80 kg; $P_{atmosphere}$ = 1010 cm H_2O; PH_2O = 63 cm H_2O; $P_{mouth(c)}$ = calibration pressure = 5.0 cm H_2O; $P_{mouth(d)}$ = calibration signal deflection in empty box = 27 mm; $P_{BOX(c)}$ = calibration volume = 30 cc; $P_{BOX(d)}$ = deflection = 49 mm; V(c) = calibration flow = 1.0 L/sec and tangent of P_{mouth}/P_{BOX} of 32° = 0.625.

Then,

$$V_{TG} = \frac{(30/49) \times (27/5.0) \times (1010 - 63) \times [530 - (80/1.07)]/530}{0.625} = 4300 \text{ mL}$$

NITROGEN WASHOUT USING OXYGEN

Theory of Measurement

The N_2 meter (or a combination of O_2 and CO_2 meters) continuously measures or calculates N_2 partial pressures or concentrations. Excluding water, the lung contains gas with approximately atmospheric concentrations of N_2 (i.e., 79%). The N_2 concentration may vary minimally, from 79% to 81%, depending on diet and degree of acute or chronic hypoventilation or hyperventilation. The intention of the test is to change the subject from breathing room air to breathing 100% O_2 while collecting all further exhaled gas until the N_2 content in the exhaled gas is very low, i.e., close to 1%.[4] The volume of collected gas times the measured concentration of N_2 should equal the volume of the lung times the initial concentration of N_2 in the lung when the directional valve was changed. It is of course necessary to know at what portion of the breathing cycle the directional valve was changed. This theoretically could be done at TLC or RV, but the change is ordinarily made at the end of a quiet exhalation, i.e., at FRC. If not turned in at FRC, it is necessary to correct the calculated volume of the lung to that at FRC. The collection is not continued indefinitely, because N_2 continues in small quantities to be washed out from body fat and to diffuse from the atmosphere into the skin, and from there to the blood and lungs. These mechanisms prevent the exhaled N_2 concentration from reaching zero percent.

Making the Measurement

The alveolar concentration of N_2 can generally be assumed to approximate 80% ($FAN_2 = 0.80$). After a subject is changed by a valve from breathing room air to breathing 100% O_2 (from a cylinder, gas bag or flexible reservoir) near the end of a quiet expiratory breath (V1), the subject continues to exhale lung gas into a flexible bag or large spirometer in which all of the exhaled gas with N_2 is collected (V2). Inhalation of O_2 is continued until the exhaled concentration of N_2 is reduced to 1.5% or less. When it reaches this level it is useful to have the subject take one or two deep breaths to wash out volumes of the lung which may not have been ventilated during quiet breathing. Generally the procedure is terminated when the end-tidal N_2 of an individual breath is reduced to 1.5% or less or after 7 minutes. In patients with moderate to severe obstructive lung disease, especially with bullae, the N_2 may be trapped and not decline to 1.5% even after several more minutes of washout. It is unreasonable to continue the washout longer than 10–12 minutes due to movement of nitrogen from fat or the surrounding air through the skin into the lung and out of the mouth into the collecting vessel. The volume and expired concentration (FEN_2) of the collected gas (V2) are measured. If the nose clip and mouthpiece are not continually sealed, N_2 may enter directly from the atmosphere, falsely increasing the concentration of N_2 and resultant calculated lung volume. If the patient has a perforated eardrum, this also will cause an inappropriate rise in N_2 concentration and lung volume. Experienced technicians suspect this when the N_2 concentration eventually does not fall and remains in the range of 2–5%. Sometimes sealing the ear canals with plugs can alleviate the inward leakage of air. An example of measurement tracings is shown in figure 6-2.

Calculations

The V_{TG} of the lung (V1 = the FRC if the valve was turned at the end of a quiet expiratory breath) $\times 0.80 = V2 \times FEN_2$. For example, with V2 of 40 L ATPS and FEN_2 of 0.04, the V1 = $40 \times 0.04/0.80 = 2.00$ L ATPS. At sea level at room temperature the factor for converting ATPS to BTPS is ~ 1.08. Thus, converting to BTPS, FRC = 2.00 $\times$ 1.08 = 2.16 L BTPS.

INERT GAS EQUILIBRATION (HELIUM)

Theory of Measurement

Helium (He) or other inert gas equilibration has been used for many decades to measure FRC, and consequently, RV and TLC.[5] Equivalently to above methods, a valve is turned to change the patient from breathing room air into a spirometer with a CO_2 absorber and a known volume of gas containing a known concentration of an insoluble gas which can be measured accurately and is not present in an appreciable concentration in room air. Hydrogen, helium or neon suffice. It is necessary for the patient to be turned into the inert gas mixture with a known percentage of inert gas at a known time in the ventilatory cycle and for the mixture to contain sufficient O_2. The patient rebreathes into the spirometer chamber while added O_2 replaces the CO_2 absorbed and the inert gas concentration has stabilized at a new lower level.[3]

Making the Measurement

A closed spirometer apparatus displays tidal volumes and helium concentrations. The apparatus contains a blower, CO_2 scrubber and at the time of switch-in, known concentrations of approximately 10% He, 21% O_2 and balance N_2. A quietly seated subject with a noseclip and mouthpiece is connected by a valve which can be switched into the spirometer at resting end-tidal expiration. While the patient rebreathes into the apparatus, O_2 is added to maintain a constant volume in the

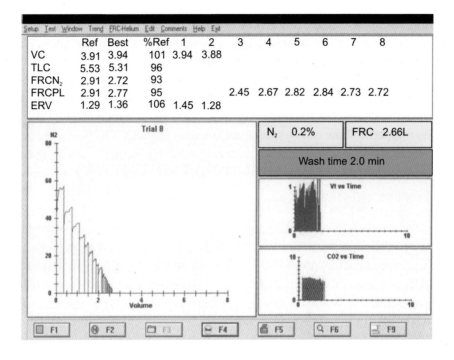

Figure 6-2 Nitrogen washout measurement of FRC. The subject has been switched from room air to 100% O_2 at the end of a normal breath. On the right, recorded against time in minutes, are tidal volumes (blue) and end-tidal CO_2 values (red). On the left N_2 concentration is recorded on the Y-axis while the calculated cumulative washed-out volume of lung from which the N_2 has been removed, breath by breath, is summed on the X-axis. In this normal subject, note the rapid decline in N_2 concentration with each successive breath. When the N_2 concentration becomes negligible (0.2% in this case), the washout was ended (2 min) while the washout volume was recorded as 2.66 L. This was corrected to an FRC of 2.72 because the "turn in" (not recorded) was not exactly at the resting end-tidal volume.

spirometer at the end of each normal tidal breath. The subject is instructed to take a deep inspiration every half-minute or so to better mix helium in the less-well-ventilated lung. After two successive such breaths show stability in end-tidal volume and He concentration, the subject is switched back from the apparatus to room air breathing. The stable He concentrations before switch-in and after switch-out are recorded for the calculations of FRC.

Calculations

$$\text{FRC + mouthpiece dead-space} = \frac{(\%He\ initial - \%He\ final) \times (V\ apparatus\ with\ added\ He + O_2)}{\%He\ final}$$

If the valve is turned at FRC, the volume of trapped lung equals the subject's FRC. If not, from observing tidal breathing on the spirometer, a correction for the larger or smaller trapped volume can be subtracted.

SINGLE BREATH EFFECTIVE ALVEOLAR VOLUME (VA')

Theory of Measurement of VA'

For relevant figures, please see Chapter 7. The single breath effective alveolar volume (VA') is measured concurrently with the diffusing capacity of the lung for carbon monoxide (DLCO), also known as the transfer factor of the lung for carbon monoxide (TLCO). Measurement of the DLCO requires that (besides sufficient O_2 and balance N_2) two key gases be inhaled concurrently.[6,7] One key gas is dilute carbon monoxide, which is avidly attracted to hemoglobin, and the other key gas is one not found in appreciable quantities in the atmosphere or lung and not absorbed nor metabolized by the lung. This inert gas is most commonly neon, helium or methane. During the single breath procedure, known concentrations of CO and inert gas are rapidly inhaled by a full inspiratory VC maneuver from RV to TLC. A shutter is then closed for 10 sec preventing the patient from exhaling. When the shutter is opened, the patient exhales rapidly so that a sample of exhaled gas can be collected and analyzed separately (for CO and Ne or He) when methane is used as the inert gas, the exhaled gas concentrations are measured continuously. In a normal patient the inert gas usually reaches at least 95% of the lung by convection and diffusion. Using the concentration and volume of the inhaled inert gas and the exhaled concentration of the inert gas allows calculation of the volume of the lung into which the inert gas was distributed (e.g., the VA'). In a patient with maldistribution of ventilation, i.e., poor distribution of the inhaled gas mixture to the entire lung, the entire lung volume is not penetrated within the 10 sec period of time.

Making the Measurement

As noted above, it is important that the patient take a full inspiratory maneuver so that the entire lung volume is exposed to the inert gas (and CO). If the inhaled inert gas is poorly distributed in the lung, due to airway obstruction or distributional differences in lung recoil, the exhaled inert gas concentration will be lower than in a normal lung of the same size and the measured VA' will be less. If the patient does not inhale to TLC, the measured VA' must also necessarily be lower. Thus, to obtain valid measures of VA' or DLCO (as the CO is distributed in the airspaces to exactly the same portions of the lung as the inert gas) the IVC volume should be as large as possible. An IVC which is 95% or more of the previously measured FVC or SVC is ideal; an IVC which is less than 90% of the previously measured FVC or SVC is usually considered unacceptable. When the measured IVC is reduced, it is usually not possible from review of the tracings to determine whether the low IVC at the start is due to incomplete exhalation to RV or incomplete inhalation to TLC (If the exhaled volume is greater than the inhaled volume, then the subject did not exhale completely at the start of the test). In order to minimize the likelihood of the patient not reaching RV before taking the full deep breath during the initial exhalation, it is important that the patient avoid taking a deep inhalation before beginning the initial exhalation to RV. This is especially true in patients with airway obstruction who take a longer time to exhale.

When methane (CH_4) is used, the exhalate can be measured continuously during the entire exhalation. When neon is used, a single sample is collected for analysis by gas chromatography. In manual systems, some experience is required in order to turn all of the valves at the correct times. In all cases, the absolute concentrations of CO and the inert gases are not critical, but the ratios of the final to the initial concentrations are critical.

Calculations

Disregarding temperature and moisture differences between inhaled and exhaled gases and lung gas, if the IVC = 3.0 L with an inhaled CH_4 fraction = 0.03% and exhaled CH_4 fraction = 0.015%, the TLC would be 6.0 L by the following equation:

$$TLC = 0.03 \times 3.0/0.015 = 6.0 \text{ L}$$

As will be discussed later, the ratio of the measured VA' to the measured TLC by plethysmography or several minutes of nitrogen washout or helium dilution is an important index of how well the inert gas in the single breath maneuver is distributed in only 10 sec. The VA'/TLC ratio is thus a good measurement of poor distribution or maldistribution of ventilation.

CHANGES IN LUNG VOLUMES WITH NORMAL AGING AND OBESITY: THE RV/VC AND IC/ERV RATIOS

As noted in Chapter 2, the TLC increases with maturation of the child and adolescent, usually reaching peak values early in the third decade. Thereafter, in the absence of extreme obesity or disease, the TLC appears to decline only minimally for the next five or six decades, in parallel with a gradual decrease in height in both men and women. As the VC declines in a near linear fashion from the end of the third decade (Figures 2-6 to 2-9 and Table 2-1), the RV increases. Admittedly, we don't often consider the RV/VC ratio, but it is of interest. Consider that the RV/VC ratio nearly doubles between ages 35 and 75 years, quite a large change. In the examples given in table 2-1, the RV/VC ratio changes from 0.35 to 0.66 in an average man and from 0.41 to 0.82 in an average woman over that time span. The decline in VC is most likely due to decreasing elastic recoil of the lung with aging, although some decrease in ventilatory muscle strength, increase in heart size and addition of intrathoracic and extrathoracic fat may also participate. It is tempting to consider the RV/TLC a more sensitive index of aging than the FRC/TLC. It would seem to be a better ratio for assessing air trapping or hyperinflation as often occurs with asthma and emphysema, but the RV is also dependent on accurate measurement of ERV.

For several decades the Harbor-UCLA pulmonary laboratories have used the recommendations found in Tables B and 30 of Comroe et al.[8] derived from publications 1948 and 1950. They state that in the sitting position, the predicted ERV is 1/3 of the VC. Unfortunately, there are no series in the last several decades which directly measure the IC and ERV from spirometry to show the influence of age and obesity on the IC and ERV. Most white populations have become more obese in the last 60 years, modifying the IC/ERV rations from those 6 decades ago. Some more recent information is available from the publication of Gutierrez et al.[9] and Quanjer et al.[10] but neither IC's nor ERV's were directly measured. From ages 20 to 80 over the usually range of heights, the predicated VC and TLC from these series do not differ markedly. In both series, one can estimate the IC's indirectly by subtracting the results of the FRC formulas from that of the TLC formulas. ERV's can be estimated indirectly by subtracting the results of the RV formulas from the FRC formulas. By examining the results using these formulas, it is evident in both series that ERV is age dependent, decreasing with age while the IC/ERV rations increase with aging. However, the IC/ERV ratios for a given age, gender, and height derived from these two series may differ from 3.9 to 2.4 or from 6.1 to 2.5 or from 2.9 to 4.7. Yet, the average differences between the IC/ERV ERV rations approximate 0.5.

The data and figure of Jones and Nzekwu[11] shed further information. They present their data as percent of predicated values using the Gutierrez et al.[9] formulas as a standard. From BMI's of 20 to 25 to BMI's of 40+, they clearly show progressively declining percent predicted values of approximately 10 to 13% in TLC, VC, and RV; 30% in FRC, and of 80% in ERV. They do not categorize data by age or present IC data or IC/ERV trends.

Using all of the above information, it can be deduced that for either men or women, the average IC/ERV ratios, IV, and ERV for ratios, IC, and ERV for ages 20 to 50 can be estimated from these three interrelated formulas:

IC/ERV $= 1.1 + 0.03 \times$ years of age, with average SD's of $<0.5'$

$IC = VC \times \dfrac{(1.1 + 0.03 \times yrs)}{(2.1 + 0.03 \times yrs)}$ and;

ERV = VC - IC.

Thus, the current approximate IC/ERV rations are as follows: 20 years = 1.7; 30 years = 2.0; 50 years = 2.6; 60 years = 2.9; 70 years = 3.2; and 80 years = 3.5.

ANALYSIS AND SELECTION OF REFERENCE EQUATIONS

Historical Perspective

For many decades the preferred equations for assessing RV and TLC were those of Goldman and Becklake.[12] This is somewhat remarkable considering that the participants selected lived at 6,000 ft land altitude in South Africa and included both smokers and non-smokers. The major reason for their continued use relates to two factors: (1) their VC measures fit well with the previous most commonly used spirometric reference equations in both men and women; and (2) they presented their data with a variety of equations so that either absolute or ratio measures could be used to match reasonably well with the values derived from the reference spirometric values reported by other authors. The lung volume equations of Crapo and his colleagues[13] also became widely used, in part because they matched very well with the spirometric and DLCO values which they had also published. They were derived from over 200 healthy never-smoking adults of Latter Day Saints living in Utah at elevations of 4000–5000 feet. A minor disadvantage was that the TLC was determined from single breath measures of 10 sec duration rather than by plethysmography or longer wash-in or wash-out techniques. However, IVC values and quality control measures were excellent, the subjects did not have significant obstructive airways disease, and radiographic TLC measurements in a large percentage of subjects were confirmatory of the VA' measurements. Thus, the VA' values they obtained should closely approximate the TLC measures that would have been found with plethysmography.

Current Perspective

For this current analysis of VC, RV and TLC lung volumes, we utilized the equations of Crapo et al.[13] and Quanjer et al.[10] from the European Steel and Coal Community, and Gutierrez et al.[11] from a large never-smoking Canadian population. We had previously compared the spirometric FVC and FEV_1 equations of Crapo et al.,[14] Gutierrez et al.,[15] Hankinson et al.,[13] J Hansen,[16] Knudson et al.,[17] Miller et al.,[18] Paoletti et al.,[19] Quanjer et al.,[10] Roca et al.[20] and the SHIP series[21] and found that

J Hansen, SHIP, Crapo, Hankinson and Miller equations were probably most representative of a white European and North American men and women.

As before, we compared the predicting formulas at 30, 50, and 70 years with heights of 185, 175, and 165 cm for men and heights of 170, 160, and 150 cm for women. To assess either lung size increase (hyperinflation or air trapping) or decrease (restriction) from predicted values, RV values rather than FRC values were used due to the lesser effect of obesity on the RV than FRC. The first point to note is that both for men and women, none of the Quanjer equations have an age factor indicating a change in TLC with age. In Gutierrez equations, the TLC slightly declines as age increases for women but remains stable for men. In the Crapo equations the TLC increases with age in men, but does not change with age in women. Looking further into the Crapo equations, it becomes apparent that in men, TLC (calculated by adding together RV and VC) results in a minor decrease in TLC with age, i.e., the opposite of the changes seen with the TLC equation alone. If we take all six series (men and women) together, the average change in TLC from age 30 to 70 is less than 5 mL/year. Overall, it seems reasonable to conclude that in health the TLC *for a given height* changes little from maturity at 20 to 25 years to 70 to 75 years, although a normal *individual's height most likely will decline by 2 to 4 centimeters with a concomitant decline in TLC in that individual.* Therefore, we will attempt to develop formulas for TLC which are stable for a given stable height. Second, regarding RV, the formulas of all four series indicate an increase in RV with age and, of course, with height. Third, in all series, the RV/TLC ratios at any age are higher in women than men.

TLC Analysis

Only a moderate agreement in TLC equation values was found in both men and women with the Crapo,[13] Gutierrez[9] and Quanjer[10] equations. Recall that for the Quanjer equations, VC values averaged over 300 mL less than mean for men and women at the nine combinations of height and age. For TLC equations, at a given height and age, differences between predicted values may exceed 0.50 L for men and 0.40 L for women while mean differences at nine typical ages and heights can average 0.39 L for men and 0.28 L for women. To finalize TLC equations which did not rely on age, the TLC equations of Crapo for men and of Gutierrez for women were revised minimally to reflect a constant TLC for the same height from ages 30 to 70 years. These equations are found in table 6-1. A new TLC equation each for men and women were derived to attempt to partially bridge these differences. Values for the new equations are closest to the predicting equations of Quanjer[10] for men and Crapo[13] for women.

"Tested at nine conditions men at ages 30, 50, and 70 and at 185, 175, and 165 cm height; women at same ages and at 170, 160, and 150 cm height."

Table 6-1	Total Lung Capacities in Men and Women. Mean Arithmetic and Absolute Differences in L Between Overall Mean Values Derived from Predicting Equations at Nine Conditions

Men	Constant (L)	Height factor (cm)	Age factor (yrs)	RSD or Syx (L)	Mean differences from new equation (L)	
					Arithmetic	Absolute
Original Crapo[13]	−7.333	0.0795	0.0032	0.792	-0.186	0.186
Modified Crapo	−7.173	0.0795			-0.186	0.186
Original Gutierrez[9]	−8.618	0.090		0.817	0.207	0.207
Original Quanjer[10]	−7.08	0.0799		0.70	-0.023	0.028
New Hansen[16]	−7.624	0.083		~ 0.75	-0.001	0.001
Women						
Original Crapo[13]	−4.537	0.0590		0.536	-0.005	0.044
Original Gutierrez[9]	−5.965	0.071	-0.007	0.583	0.137	0.151
Modified Gutierrez	−6.31	0.071			0.142	0.142
Original Quanjer[10]	−5.79	0.066		0.060	-0.138	0.138
New Hansen[16]	−5.545	0.06533		~ 0.55	0.000	0.000

RV/TLC Analysis

We also added a composite of RV/TLC for each gender, each of which results in the smallest deviations from the original equations of Crapo, Gutierrez, and Quanjer et al.[9,10,13] These results are shown in figure 6-3 and table 6-2. There are reasonably good, not excellent, agreements between these series. A composite equation (Mean)[16] is given in table 6-2 which yields reasonable values for RV/TLC and TLC values using the recommended FVC equations from Chapter 4.

RV Analysis

After checking many combinations of absolute VC, RV, TLC values and their ratios, the tightest agreement was found with the Crapo, Gutierrez, and Quanjer et al.[9,10,13] equations for RV. In addition separate new equations for RV for men and women are

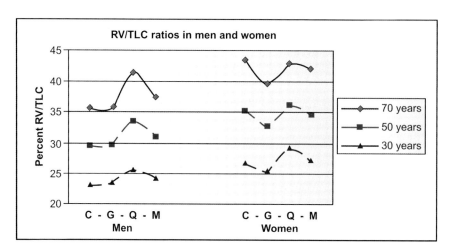

Figure 6-3 Residual volume/total lung capacity ratios (RV/TLC) in percent for men and women using the original Crapo (C), Gutierrez (G) and Quanjer (Q) et al.[9,10,13] predicting equations. For each gender, the mean values found using each of the other three gender-specific equations are identified as mean (M).

Table 6-2	Residual Volume/Total Lung Capacity (RV/TLC) Predicting Equations for Men and Women from Three Series (Crapo, Gutierrez, and Quanjer et al.[9,10,13]) with Their Predicted RV/TLC Values at 30, 50, and 70 years. RSD = 5.5% for Men and 5.1% for Women. New (Mean) Derived Equation Added[16]

MEN				RV/TLC values (percent)	
Author	Constant (percent)	Age	30 yr	50 yr	70 yr
Crapo	14.06	0.309	23.3	29.5	35.7
Gutierrez	14.6	0.30	23.6	29.6	35.6
Quanjer	14	0.39	25.7	33.5	41.3
Mean	14.22	0.333	24.2	30.9	37.5

Consequently, for men, from last equation, predicted VC/TLC = 0.8578 – 0.00333 × age; predicted TLC = predicted VC/(0.8578 – 0.00333 × years of age)[16]

WOMEN		Age	30 yr	50 yr	70 yr
Crapo	14.35	0.416	26.8	35.2	43.5
Gutierrez	15.1	0.35	25.6	32.6	39.6
Quanjer	19	0.34	29.2	36	42.8
Mean	16.15	0.369	27.2	34.6	42.0

Consequently, for women, from last equation, predicted VC/TLC = 0.8385 – 0.00369 × age; predicted TLC = predicted VC/(0.8385 – 0.00369 × years of age)[16]

presented. The values from each of these equations equal the average values of the RV at all nine heights and ages. The mean or composite formula for women is: RV (L) = -2.258 + 0.0193 × cm + 0.017 × years. The formula for men is: RV (L) = -2.164 + 0.0182 × cm + 0.0212 × years.[16] Figures 6-4A and B show the deviations from these formulas of the values derived from the original equations of Crapo, Gutierrez and

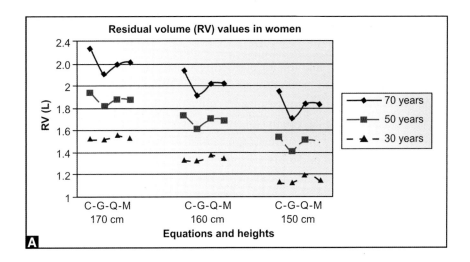

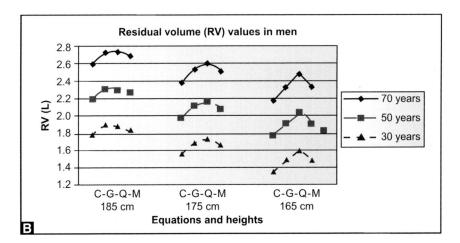

Figures 6-4A and B Residual volume (RV) values obtained using RV formulas of Crapo et al (C), Gutierrez et al (G), Quanjer et al (Q)[9,10,13] as well as those of a new mean formula (M) in: (A) women: RV (L) = -2.258 + 0.0193 × cm + 0.017 × years and (B) men: RV (L) = -2.164 + 0.0182 x cm + 0.0212 × years[16]

Quanjer et al. The average deviations from the new equations at the nine conditions of height and age were 71 mL for men and 50 mL for women.

We found that using these new RV equations with six series of VC values from Chapter 4 gave us quite consistent values for RV, VC and TLC for both men and women, more consistent than with any other combination of formulas. The mean SDs for RV, VC and TLC for these six series with four combinations of height and age (150 and 170 cm for women and 165 and 185 cm for men at ages 30 and 70 years) were 50 mL for women and 79 mL for men (Figures 6-5 and 6-6).

Summary of Lung Volume Findings

There is no single perfect solution for predicting RV, TLV and RV/TLC ratios. There are limited series of recent predicting equations for RV and TLC to deal with, and they lead to somewhat conflicting results. It is quite possible, for populations in good health, that TLC values for a given height rise with age or that they decline minimally with age. The mean RSD or SEE of the Crapo, Gutierrez and Quanjer sets of equations for RV are 0.418 L for men and 0.370 L for women. Presumably the RSD for the new RV equations are similar so 95% confidence limits are $0.418 \times 1.645 = 0.688$ L for men and $0.370 \times 1.645 = 0.608$ L for women. In these series measuring TLC, the RSD or SEE averages were 0.770 L for men and 0.573 L for women, yielding 95% confidence

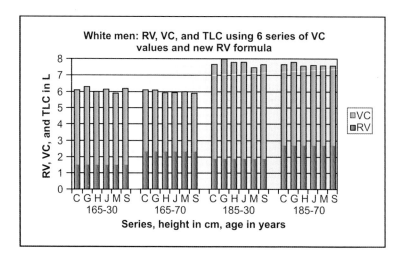

Figure 6-5 Values of RV for white men from a new formula (RV in L = -2.164 + 0.0182 x cm + 0.0212 x years)[16] plus VC values from six series of formulas (Crapo = C, Gutierrez = G, Hankinson = H, J Hansen = J, Miller = M and SHIP = S)[9,14-16,18,21] at four conditions (two heights and two ages). The RV + VC values give quite consistent TLC values for each condition across the six series

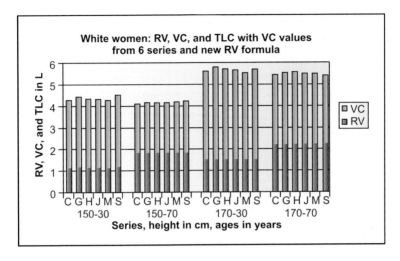

Figure 6-6 Values of RV for white women from a new formula (RV in L = -2.258 + 0.0193 x cm + 0.017 x years) plus VC values from six series of formulas (Crapo = C, Gutierrez = G, Hankinson = H, J Hansen = J, Miller = M and SHIP = S)[9,14-16,18,21] at four conditions (two heights and two ages). The RV + VC values give quite consistent TLC values for each condition across the six series

limits of ±1.266 L for men and ±0.943 L for women from mean predicted values. In both men and women, the variability between series increased with lung volumes larger than average (taller and younger) and decreased with lung volumes lower than average(shorter and older) so that the one-tailed 95% confidence limits for all situations averaged 119% and 81% of mean predicted for women and 120% and 80% of mean predicted for men. Thus, it seems reasonable to consider that TLC values within 80% to 120% of mean predicted values are likely to be within normal limits and those outside these limits are not likely to be within normal limits.

The report of Garcia-Rio et al.[22] of Spanish adults in apparent excellent health from age 65 to 85 years casts some doubt on the changes in lung volumes after age 65. They measured lung volumes by both plethysmography and helium dilution and found RV volumes averaged approximately 230 mL more in men and 90 mL more in women by plethysmography. By either method, using their published height and age coefficients, they reported unchanging values of RV in both men and women from age 65 to 85. Other studies (Gutierrez) with equal or greater number of subjects from age 60 to 80 found increases of approximately 300 mL in RV in women and 400 mL in men over that same time period. Moreover, Garcia-Rio et al. found decreases in VC of 680 mL in women and 950 mL in men over the same time frame while VC decreases in the Crapo, Gutierrez and Quanjer series over the same time frame were only 420–520 mL in both women and men. As

TLC = VC + RV, TLC over 20 years in the Garcia-Rio series decreased an average of 1,100 mL in women and 1,000 mL in men while Crapo, Quanjer and Gutierrez series each found decreases of only 100–200 mL in women and 0–100 mL in men. These greater declines in VC, RV and TLC in Garcia-Rio series could lead one to rely predominantly on the other three series, although the matter probably remains in dispute. However, there is no dispute that RV/TLC values increase in every series as their population ages.

Undeniably, RV universally increases with age, and men's and women's RV/TLC differ slightly. In addition to the minor variability in mean predicted values, the large RSD or SEE in each series of equations discloses the large variability within the population sampled in each series. This *within series variability far exceeds the between series variability*. Consequently, as with all timed volume measurements, caution should be used in assessing deviations from mean predicted values. Nevertheless, the concordance between series using the new RV equations' values is somewhat reassuring.

Since concordance between series for TLC seems to be best achieved by using RV equations for white women and men, the following equations are recommended: For women:

$$RV\,(L) = -2.258 + 0.0193 \times cm + 0.017 \times years.$$

For men:

$$RV\,(L) = -2.164 + 0.0182 \times cm + 0.0213 \times years.$$

If these RV values are added to the predicted FVC values derived from the recommended equations in Chapter 4, the resultant predicted FVC, RV and TLC values are reasonable to use in laboratory reports and interpretations. Dividing this predicted RV by this predicted TLC yields an appropriate predicted RV/TLC.

ANALYZING CHANGES IN LUNG SIZE

Lung Size within 95% Confidence Limits: Caution

Since the considerable variability in lung size among normal individuals of the same gender, age, height and ethnicity, one should be cautious in positively identifying changes in TLC as due to restriction or hyperinflation, unless the decrease or increase in measured TLC is clearly greater than the one-tailed 95% confidence limits. Importantly, almost every disorder listed in the immediately following sections as a cause of lung restriction or hyperinflation may be present in an individual and NOT cause a statistically significant change in lung volumes. However, if there are prior measurements of lung volume in a given individual, a reduction of 8–10% from prior values of TLC should be outside the range of day-to-day variability or laboratory error. It is reasonable for a physician who does not know the patient but who interprets the tests to suggest diagnoses without expressing certainty. But, for example, primary pulmonary hypertension may be far advanced without statistically significant changes in spirometry, lung size or even DLCO.

Decreases in Lung Size

Restriction is defined as a reduction in TLC. Since a reduction in VC may be due to either obstructive or restrictive lung disease, it is important not to identify all reductions in VC as restriction. Marked reductions in VC are common in obstructive lung disease and should not be considered evidence of restriction. The pattern of an FEV_1 and FVC below the LLN but with a normal FEV_1/FVC is suggestive but not diagnostic of restrictive disease, especially when the FEV_1/FVC is low normal or borderline abnormal.

Restriction may be due to intrinsic lung disease or extrinsic factors, i.e. outside the lung proper. Sometimes both intrinsic and extrinsic factors are present. Considering intrinsic restrictive lung disease first, the percentage reduction in VC is often greater than the reduction in RV, although each may be similarly reduced. Solitary reduction in RV without a decrease in VC is unusual and suggests the possibility of measurement error.

The term "lung restriction" rather than "restrictive lung disease" seems appropriate to use when the lung size is reduced only by extrinsic factors. Thus, cardiomegaly, lymph node enlargement, chest wall disease, some malignancies, diaphragmatic paralysis and weakness can be considered cause of lung restriction. In these cases when disorders are within the lung, the term "restrictive lung disease" is appropriate. Pleural effusion, empyema and pneumothorax all cause reduction in aerated lung volume and can be considered both intrinsic and extrinsic. The laboratory diagnosis of pneumothorax can be challenging. If the pneumothroax is of adequate size, TLC measured by nitrogen washout or helium dilution will be decreased while TLC measured by plethysmography will be increased.

The most common cause of lung restriction seen in our clinical laboratory is obesity. Unless accompanied by heart failure, this is an extrinsic factor and does not usually warrant the term "restrictive lung disease", but is more properly called "lung restriction". The PFT pattern of obesity is usually obvious.[23] Classically, the ERV is considerably reduced and the IC/ERV ratio elevated above 2:1 or 3:1, and may be even 10:1 or more. If: (1) the IC is three-fourth or more of the predicted IC; (2) the VC and TLC are only reduced as much as the ERV is reduced and (3) there is no evidence airway obstruction (normal FEV_1/FVC) and/or loss of pulmonary vasculature (normal DLCO), this pattern can nearly always safely be attributed exclusively to obesity. If FEV_1/FVC or DLCO are abnormal or the lung volumes are further reduced, additional diagnoses must be strongly entertained. When obesity is very severe (BMI > 40) then further reduction in IC, VC, RV and TLC can be due to obesity alone or due to heart failure or other added disorders.

Other common and uncommon disorders which often (but not always) cause restrictive lung disease are: pneumonias of any cause; pulmonary fibrosis; neoplasms; atelectasis; silicosis, asbestosis, other pneumoconiosis and sarcoidosis; all of the autoimmune rheumatologic diseases; heart failure, pulmonary edema or infarcts; radiation fibrosis; drug reactions; acute respiratory distress syndrome; alveolar proteinosis; cystic fibrosis, bronchiectasis, and others.

Increases in Lung Size

Approximately 5% of individuals (included in a reference population of a given age, gender, ethnicity and height) have lung volumes that are above the statistically determined one-tailed confidence limits of VC and TLC. If these findings are accompanied by near-normal or normal DLCO and no evidence of airway obstruction, these individuals are likely to really be "above normal" and not abnormal. However, if the FEV_1/FVC or FEV_3/FVC is decreased or the RV/TLC ratio increased, or the DLCO and DLCO/VA are borderline or abnormal, then that individual likely has obstructive airways disease.

Classically, individuals with obstructive lung disease predominantly have asthma, bronchitis, emphysema or any combination of these three disorders. To complicate the issue, they may also have pulmonary fibrosis or other disorders. In an acute asthma attack, lung volume may be reduced due to atelectasis or lung volume may be increased due to marked hyperinflation. Typically, if hyperinflated, the RV is increased more than the TLC indicating air trapping. Typically, chronic bronchitis alone is not accompanied by hyperinflation; with emphysema, the TLC and especially the RV are nearly always elevated. The DLCO and DLCO/VA measurements are helpful in discriminating. Patients with cystic fibrosis, bronchiectasis and some pneumoconioses can also have obstructive lung disease with destroyed lung with or without bullae. When reviewing nitrogen washout tracings in individuals with bullae or very poorly emptying airspaces, one may see one or more blips in N_2 concentration during the washout process. It is likely to occur when the individual is coached to take a deep breath which, in the absence of a mouthpiece leak, is typical of the emptying of a previously poorly communicating bullous lesion.

REFERENCES

1. Comroe, JH. Retrospectoscope: Man-Cans. *Amer Rev Resp Dis*. 1977;116:945-50.
2. DuBois AB, Botelho SY, Bedell GN, et al. A rapid plethysmographic method for measuring thoracic gas volume. *J Clin Invest*. 1956;35:322-6.
3. Clausen JL (Ed). Pulmonary Function Testing Guidelines and Controversies: Equipment, Methods, and Normal Values. New York: Academic Press; 1982. pp. 1-365.

4. Darling RC, Cournand A, Richards DW Jr. Studies on the intrapulmonary mixture of gases. III. An open circuit method for measuring residual air. *J Clin Invest*. 1940;19:609-18.

5. Meneely GR, Ball CO, Kory RC, et al. A simplified closed circuit helium dilution method for the determination of the residual volume of the lungs. *Am J Med*. 1960;28:824-31.

6. MacIntyre N, Crapo RO, Viegi DC, et al. Standardization of the single-breath determination of carbon monoxide uptake in the lung. *Eur Respir J*. 2005;26:720-35.

7. Ogilvie CM, Forster RE, Blackemore WS, et al. A standardized breath holding technique for the clinical measurement of diffusing capacity of the lung for carbon monoxide. *J Clin Invest*. 1957;36:1-17.

8. Comroe JH Jr, Forster RE II, DuBois AB, Briscoe WA, Carlsen E. The Lung: Clinical Physiology and Pulmonary Function Tests, 2nd ed. year book, Chicago 2004.

9. Gutierrez C, Ghezzo RH, Abboud RT, Cosio MG, et al. References values of pulmonary function test for Canadian Caucasians. *Can Respir J*. 2004;11:414-24.

10. Quanjer PH, Tammiling GJ, Cotes JE, et al Lung volumes and forced expiratory flows. Report Working Party Standardization of Lung Function Tests, European Community for Steel and Coal. Official Statement of the European Respiratory Society. *Eur Respir J*. 1993;(6)16:15-40.

11. Jones rL, Nzekwu M-M, The effects of body mass index on lung volumes. *Chest*. 2006; 130: 827-33.

12. Goldman HI, Becklake MR. Respiratory function tests. Normal values at median altitudes and the prediction of normal results. *Amer Rev Tuberc*. 1959;79:457-67.

13. Crapo RO, Morris AH, Clayton PD, et al. Lung volumes in healthy nonsmoking adults. *Bull Eur Physiopathol Respir*. 1982;18:419-25.

14. Crapo RO, Morris AH, Gardner RM. Reference spirometric values using techniques and equipment that meet ATS requirements. *Am Rev Respir Dis*. 1981;123:659-64.

15. Hankinson JL, Odenkranz JR, Fedan KB. Spirometric reference values from a sample of the general U.S. population. *Am J Respir Crit Care Med*. 1999;159:179-87.

16. Hansen JE. Unpublished observations.

17. Knudson RJ, Lebowitz MD, Holberg CJ. Changes in the normal maximal expiratory flow-volume curve with growth and aging. *Am Rev Respir Dis*. 1983;127:725-34.

18. Miller MR, Grove DM, Pincock AC. Time domain spirogram indices. Their variability and reference values in nonsmokers. *Am Rev Respir Dis*. 1985;132:1041-8.

19. Paoletti P, Pistelli G, Fazzi P, et al. Reference values for vital capacity and flow volume curves from a general population study. *Bull Eur Physiolathol Respir*. 1986;22:451-9.

20. Roca J, Sanchis J, Agusti-Videl A, et al. Spirometric reference values for a Mediterranean population. *Bull Europ Physiopathol Respir*. 1986;22:451-9.

21. Koch B, Schäper C, Ittermann T, et al. Reference values for lung function testing in adults—results from the study of health in Pomerania (SHIP). *Dtsch Med Wochenschr*. 2009;134:2327-32.

22. Garcia-Rio F, Dorgham A, Pino JM, et al. Lung volume reference values for women and men 65 to 85 years of age. *Am J Respir Crit Care Med*. 2009;180:1083-91.

23. Ray CS, Sue DY, Bray G, et al. Effects of obesity on respiratory function. *Am Rev Resp Dis*. 1983;128:510-6.

Single-Breath DLCO, TLCO, DLCO/VA' and VA' Measures More than Diffusion

INTRODUCTION AND HISTORY

The measurement of the single-breath transfer factor for carbon monoxide (TLCO) or, as it is alternately and less appropriately named, the diffusing capacity for carbon monoxide (DLCO) is important, interesting and useful in assessing lung disease. To minimize confusions we will use in this chapter, the most frequently used abbreviation, i.e., DLCO. Diffusion is the mechanism which transports molecules around a mixture dependent on random Brownian movement. In 1855, Adolf Fick formulated two laws of diffusion. These laws state that molecules move from regions of high concentrations to regions of low concentration proportional to the differences in concentrations. Further, as concentration differences decrease over time, movement between areas of differing concentrations slows. When concentrations differ markedly, movement is rapid. When membranes are involved, diffusion is dependent on permeability, solubility, concentration differences, time, area, and temperature. Since it was not technically possible to measure movement of O_2 from the atmosphere to the red cells in the pulmonary capillaries, measuring the transfer of CO rather than O_2 from the atmosphere to the pulmonary capillary was substituted because the concentration of CO in the red cells was almost negligible.

The transfer of CO from inhaled gas can be measured either at rest or during exercise. A century ago, Marie Krogh and colleagues measured the transfer of CO at rest using a single-breath technique with hydrogen as a tracer gas.[1] Riley and Filley and their colleagues[2,3] developed techniques to measure CO uptake during exercise, but these techniques are now rarely used due to their complexity and the necessity of arterial blood analyses. Fowler and Roughton[4] added theoretical knowledge and data regarding the diffusion of gases in the air, tissues and blood. In the late 1950s, Shepard, Ogilvie, Burrows and their colleagues[5-7] developed and began to utilize a single-breath method using CO and an inert "tracer" gases other than hydrogen. They laid the groundwork establishing the clinical importance of the single-breath measurement of CO transfer. Now, the simple single-breath technique has been standardized so that the transfer of CO during exercise is rarely measured. Excluding spirometry, it has become the single most important test in clinically evaluating lung function. Before going further into the necessary calculation and interpretation, let's examine the testing equipment and the procedure.

EQUIPMENT AND PROCEDURE

Equipment

It is always desirable to carefully read and follow the manufacturer's instructions regarding the device, calibrations, procedures, directions, quality control procedures, cautions, and directions. The required equipment includes a way to record and measure the speed and quantity of inspired volume, the duration of breath-holding and the timing of collection of the expired gases during the alveolar phase, i.e., after the equipment and large airway dead space has been cleared. It must allow: (a) switching from room air into a gas mixture with about 21% O_2 (or slight enrichment at altitude) and smaller quantities of CO (usually 0.3%) and a tracer gas; (b) forced breath-holding for about 10 seconds; (c) accurate measurement of the concentrations of expired gases during the alveolar phase, and (d) comparison with the inspired concentrations of gases. Both self-fabricated and commercial systems must allow this. Although the exact fractions of the inhaled and alveolar gases need not be known, the gas analyzers must be inherently linear or software linearized across the range of inspired to alveolar partial pressures. Equipment dead space should be minimal and known (Figure 7-1).

Procedure

The patient must be comfortably seated with a nose clip, coached to make a complete exhalation to RV through the mouthpiece, coached to inhale to TLC and breath-hold for about 10 seconds, and then allowed to exhale rapidly while a discrete alveolar or continuous sample of gases is collected. If discrete samples of inhaled and exhaled gas are analyzed, there is only one chance (requiring good coordination by the technician) to collect the exhaled gases during the "alveolar plateau." Thus the technician must be very familiar with the equipment and well skilled. When the patient has a reduction in VC near 1.0 L or less, it may or may not be possible to collect valid samples. After 2-3 minutes allow washout of the tracer gas, the test can be repeated. Generally no more than three tests are done at one sitting. Due to the increase in blood COHb of approximately 1% per test, the measured DLCO declines with repetitive testing by about 1% per test.

With good cooperation and properly performed methods, two samples usually agree within 10%. If not, a 3rd measurement, and rarely a 4th measurement may be done. Hopefully, the inspired VC equals or exceeds 90% of the VC measured earlier that day. If the IVC is less than 90% of the best FVC, the values need not be discarded,

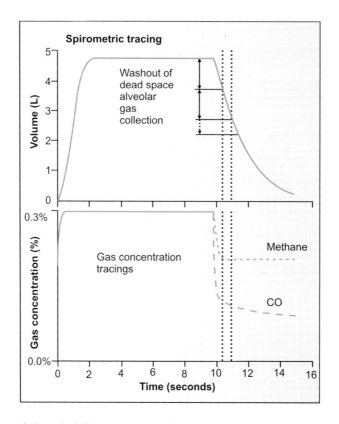

Figure 7-1 Single-breath diffusing capacity of the lung (DLCO). The top half of the figure shows a spirometric tracing of: (1) initial full rapid inhalation to total lung capacity; (2) breath-holding for 10 seconds because the valve allowing exhalation is closed and (3) opening of the valve with exhalation and collection of alveolar sample after dead space washout. The full exhalation before the initial full inhalation is not recorded. The bottom half of the figure shows the recordings of CO and methane (CH_4) from continuous gas analyzers. The initial concentration of CO and (CH_4) are both 0.3% (top of tracing), recorded while the closed valve prevents the patient from exhaling. During exhalation the gas concentrations fall quickly. After the washout of the equipment and airway deadspace, the concentrations of CH_4 are quite stable while the concentration of CO gradually declines. Using continuous gas analyzers, one can shift the "collection time" to earlier or later in exhalation. The resultant calculated values for DLCO and effective alveolar volume (VA') vary minimally. When non-continuous gas analyzers (Ne or He and CO are used, a timed alveolar sample is collected during exhalation between the two vertical dotted lines or shortly thereafter) after dead space washout is complete. Inert gas concentrations are used to calculate VA' while ratios of all gases are used to calculate DLCO values. Only ratios rather than absolute concentrations of inhaled and exhaled gas concentrations of the gases are necessary for measurements and calculations.

but they are more difficult to interpret. Generally, the value with the highest or higher IVC will also include the highest or higher DLCO. If the IVC values are lower than 90% of the previously measured best VC, it is usually impossible to say whether that is a result of incomplete expiration or incomplete inspiration. However, if tracings show that the expired volume exceeds the inspired volume, the error can be attributed to an initial incomplete expiration.

There is no infallible rule as to what measurement(s) to finally report. Measurements from a single maneuver can be accepted, but it is preferable to average the two highest values for VA' and DLCO. Because errors in measured concentrations of both CO and CH_4 (or other inert gas) can be higher or lower than true values, the DLCO and concurrent VA' values should be averaged if they differ by less than 10%. If in doubt, the technician should review all recordings, select the one, two or three tracings and values that appear most likely to represent the patient's best efforts, and report his or her degree of uncertainty to the physician interpreting the test.

THEORY AND CALCULATIONS

VA'

The addition of the tracer gas allows not only the measurement of DLCO' but also the measurement of the VA' which is the volume of the lung exposed to the tracer gas and CO during the 10-second breath hold. The tracer gas must be almost or completely insoluble in water and tissue during the 10-second breath hold. Commonly used tracer gases are helium (He), neon (Ne) and CH_4. This tracer gas serves the important function of allowing the calculation of the effective volume of lung, i.e., the lung volume into which the tracer gas and CO were diluted during the 10-second breath-holding period. Examples: (1) If inhaled Ne = 0.3%, inspired VC (IVC) = 4.0 L, and exhaled Ne = 0.2%; then VA' = 4 × 0.3/0.2 = 6 L. (2) If inhaled Ne = 0.3%, IVC = 2.8 L, and exhaled Ne = 0.24%; then VA' = 2.8 × 0.3/0.24 = 3.5 L.

In normal individuals the inhaled tracer gas reaches over 95% of the entire lung airspaces within the 10-second breath-hold. Thus, in an individual without airway obstruction or maldistribution of ventilation and completing a full inhalation from RV to TLC, this effective alveolar volume or VA is 95-100% of the individual's actual TLC. It may not equal the TLC because a small correction of ~0.2 L should be made for the equipment and upper airways "dead space." If the initial "full" inhalation is less than 90% of the known VC, the test is inferior. With such a poor inhalation, it is difficult to determine whether the reduced inhalation is due to an initial incomplete exhalation to RV or to a lack of full inhalation to TLC.

VA'/TLC

In a patient population (i.e., not known if normal or abnormal) the determination of the VA' to the measured TLC (by plethysmography, N_2 washout or He equilibration) is valuable. If the VA' was determined from an IVC greater than 90% of the known best VC, and gas ratios were properly measured, then the ratio of VA'/TLC is a measurement of the 10-second volume distribution of an inert gas (VA')/to the volume distribution during longer washout or equilibration (TLC). Thus a low VA/TLC discloses poor distribution or maldistribution of ventilation. From a practical viewpoint, a VA'/TLC less than 85% should be considered abnormal indicating maldistribution of ventilation. If, perhaps, the VA' exceeds the TLC by more than 10%, there likely is some procedural, measurement or calculation error in the measurement of either VA' or the components of the TLC.

DLCO

With bulk flow or ventilation, all gases, such as CO_2, O_2, N_2, H_2O, and CO, flow or move together, in and out with each breath, from the mouth to the respiratory bronchioles and perhaps proximal alveolar ducts. With diffusion of gases due to Brownian movement, whether in gas, liquid or tissue, the molecules move in differing directions from one space to another, depending on the concentration or partial pressure differences of each gas between these spaces, the solubility of the gases, and whatever barriers there may be to their movement. Within the gaseous airspaces of the normal acini distal to the respiratory bronchioles (i.e., in alveolar ducts, sacs and alveoli), there is no normal barrier to gaseous diffusion, only the limitation of time to move O_2, CO, CO_2, N_2 and the rare gases. The distance to the alveolar capillaries from the alveolar ducts for gaseous transport is shorter than was previously estimated (Chapter 2).

The amount of CO that is transferred from the airspaces to the hemoglobin in the capillaries is dependent on six factors: (1) ventilation; (2) gas concentrations; (3) perfusion; (4) hemoglobin; (5) time, and (6) fluids, debris or fibrosis in the airspaces. First, the inhaled CO must be ventilated to the acinus. Second, the difference in partial pressures between O_2 or CO in the airspaces and the red cell (Partial pressure is proportional to concentration). Third, the airspaces in the acinus must have capillaries with blood, i.e., perfusion. Fourth, the capillaries must have quantities of normal reduced hemoglobin able to accept the CO. This quantity is reduced in anemia, carboxyhemoglobinemia, or when perfusion through the pulmonary capillaries is markedly delayed. Fifth, the movements of O_2 and CO are dependent on time. Thus all of these six factors affect the transfer of O_2 or CO from inhaled gas to the red cell during a 10-second breath hold. Sixth, edema fluid, debris in the alveoli or fibrosis of the alveoli may slow the movement of O_2 or CO, i.e., diffusion. Although this entire transfer is more appropriately identified as "transfer factor of the lung" since so much more than diffusion is involved we will use the abbreviation of DLCO to reduce confusion with the abbreviation TLC. Regardless of the nomenclature, all of the six factors listed affect the results of the informative single-breath DLCO. Clinically, slow diffusion through fibrotic membranes is uncommonly the cause of a low DLCO! Other factors are usually responsible.

The proper timing of the exposure of inspired CO to the pulmonary airspaces has been debated, since inhalation and exhalation are not instantaneous but take some time. Figure 7-2 demonstrates the three most common ways that the time of exposure has been calculated. Each one could be justified as reasonable; however, the current consensus is to use the Jones-Meade method of timing the breath-holding time.[8]

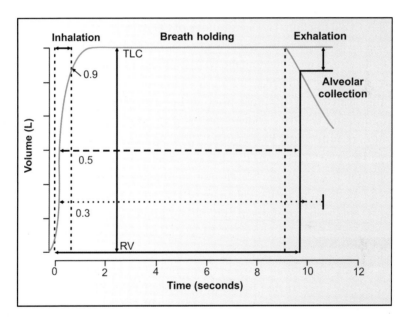

Figure 7-2 Three alternative methods of timing the breath-holding period for the single-breath tests. Inhalation time is considered to be from the back-extrapolated onset on inhalation to 90% of the complete inhalation. The original Ogilvie method[6] (solid horizontal line) measures from the back-extrapolated onset of inhalation to the beginning of the sample collection. The Jones-Meade method[8] (dotted horizontal line) measures from 30% of the back-extrapolated onset of inhalation time to mid-time of the sample collection. The Epidemiologic Standardization Project method[9] (dashed horizontal line) measures from 50% of the back-extrapolated inhalation time to the start of the sample collection. The Jones-Meade method is currently recommended.[10] (RV = residual volume; TLC = total lung capacity)

The units of measurement for DLCO are: mL/min/mmHg or mmol/min/kPa. The VA is measured as L, BTPS but is converted to STPD in the equation below. The calculations require the measurement of time, barometric pressure, IVC (inspired volume) and the ratio of concentrations of inhaled CO and tracer gas (Ne, CH_4 or He) and exhaled alveolar CO and tracer gas. There are minor differences as to how the exposure time is measured. The most commonly used Jones-Meade method measures time between ~1/3 of the inhalation time and the mid-collection time of the alveolar gas. The exact concentration of CO and Ne are not required, only their relative concentrations in the following equation:

$$\text{DLCO (mL/min/mmHg)} = \frac{\text{VA}'(\text{STPD}) \times 60}{(\text{PB-47}) \times t} \times \log_e \frac{(F_I CO_0 \times F_E Ne)}{(F_A CO_t \times F_I Ne)}$$

Where PB = barometric pressure; t = time in seconds; $\log_e$ = natural logarithm; $F_I CO_0$ and $F_A CO_t$ = fractional concentrations of CO in inspired and expired alveolar gases; and $F_I Ne$ and $F_E Ne$ = fractional inspired and expired concentrations of Ne or other insoluble tracer gas. Dividing the DLCO values in mL/min/mmHg by 3.0 gives DLCO values in mmol/min/kPa.

Since the transfer of CO decreases as the difference between alveolar gas concentrations and capillary concentrations decrease during the breath-holding, the logarithm of time to the base is used. With equipment that allows flexibility in the timing of breath-holding one can test the validity of the measurement of DLCO by shortening or extending the breath-holding time to perhaps 6 or 20 seconds. In doing so, one finds quite similar calculated DLCO values, confirming the reliability of the theory, equations, equipment and measurement techniques.

DLCO/VA' and KCO

As noted before, the inhaled tracer gas and CO concentrations are equally distributed to the lung so that the ratio of inhaled/exhaled concentration of the tracer gas measures the VA'. It does not measure the TLC, except in patients with good tests, normal compliance and without airway obstruction or maldistribution of ventilation. Thus, the DLCO/VA' or KCO can be easily calculated in the units of mL/min/mmHg (STPD)/VA' (BTPS).

INTERPRETING THE RATIOS

VA'/TLC

In an individual known to be normal with a good technique and measurement of IVC and inhaled and exhaled alveolar Ne, one can properly measure VA' and thus TLC. In patients, however, VA' does not necessarily equal TLC. If one has a valid measure of TLC by another method, i.e., radiographic, plethysmographic, nitrogen washout or helium dilution, and a valid measure of VA' one can easily calculate the proportional volume of lung reached in the 10-second breath-hold. Example: If TLC is 8 L by plethysmography and VA' is 6 L by single-breath DLCO measurement, then only about 75% of the lung was reached by the He and only about 75% of the lung was reached by the CO. This tells us that there was no distribution of either He or CO to 25% of the lung and therefore, significant maldistribution is present.

DLCO/VA' and KCO

The ratio of DLCO/VA', which is the same as the TLCO/VA' or transfer *coefficient*, is also identified as the KCO. It is reasonable to think of the KCO as the alveolar *concentration* of capillaries with hemoglobin-containing red cells in the lung ventilated during the single-breath maneuver. As DLCO/VA' does not measure the transfer of CO in volumes of the lung that were not measured by the single-breath maneuver, it is wrong to extrapolate the DLCO/VA' to the remainder of the lung.

Admittedly there are occasions when the pulmonary alveolar capillaries are not destroyed, but are present and contain blood resulting in a low KCO or DLCO/VA', but these situations are infrequent. Examples of these occasions are pulmonary edema, alveolar proteinosis, pneumocystis pneumonia, and pulmonoary fibrosis. In the former three, alveolar filling with fluid may inhibit the CO reaching the capillaries. With pulmonary fibrosis, it is most likely that the pulmonary capillaries have really been destroyed and DLCO/VA, may not improve with time. However, most commonly, DLCO/VA' is dependent on continuing lung capillary perfusion and the availability of hemoglobin.

Some Examples

Assume four patients, each with normal hemoglobin of 15 g/100 mL a predicted DLCO of 30 mL/min/mmHg and a predicted TLC of 6 L. Their predicted DLCO/VA' is 30/6 or 5.0 (Table 7-1).

Patient #1 has low VA'/TLC. The low VA'/TLC of 4/6 = 67% means there is maldistribution of ventilation. The DLCO and DLCO/VA' are reduced, especially the DLCO. Overall gas transfer is reduced. Within the lung volumes reached by the inert gas, the DLCO/VA' is also reduced, meaning either that the number of pulmonary capillaries are reduced or that perfusion of the ventilated lung is reduced or both. What can one say about the capillary density in the lung not reached by the inert gas? Nothing, this volume is silent. This is one of the patterns that may be seen in congestive heart failure.

Patient #2 has a low TLC and low VA' with a ratio of 100%. This is restrictive lung disease. One cannot expect the VA' to be appreciably larger than the TLC unless

Table 7-1	Hypothetical Patients, Each with a Hemoglobin of 15 g/100 mL Blood, with Predicted Values of TLC of 6 L, DLCO of 30 mL/min/mmHg and DLCO/VA' of 5. Their Actual Values of TLC, VA' and DLCO Differ			
Patient #	Measured TLC (L)	Measured VA' (L)	Measured DLCO (mL/min/mmHg)	Measured DLCO/VA'
1	6.0	4.0	16.0	4.0
2	4.0	4.0	16.0	4.0
3	8.0	6.0	12.0	2.0
4	6.0	6.0	16.0	2.7

there are measurement errors. The DLCO and DLCO/VA' are also reduced indicating some destruction of capillaries or extensive fibrosis or alveolar filling in the lung.

Patient #3 has an elevated TLC, maldistribution of ventilation (VA'/TLC = 6/8 = 75%), low DLCO and even lower DLCO/VA'. Reduction in FEV_1/FVC is very likely. This pattern, with hyperinflation and destroyed pulmonary capillaries, fits emphysema well.

Patient #4 has a normal TLC and VA', but a low DLCO and an even lower DLCO/VA' (DLCO/VA' = 2.7/5.0 = 54%). This is not maldistribution or restriction, but is destruction or non-availability of alveolar capillaries. If there were no airway obstruction this would be very suggestive of pulmonary vascular disease.

"Correcting" for Carboxyhemoglobinemia, Anemia, and Erythrocythemia

One can also make repeated measurements of DLCO every 5 minutes in the same normal individual for 10 or more times. In doing so, one finds a reduction of about 1% in DLCO after each maneuver and a rise in venous carboxyhemoglobin (COHgb) of 10%. This is important for two theoretical reasons: First, an increase in COHgb reduces the DLCO proportionally. Second, it indicates that the volume of reduced hemoglobin entering the pulmonary capillaries affects the uptake of CO and the DLCO. Thus, there must be some dependence of measured DLCO on the perfusion of quantity of non COHgb into the pulmonary capillaries.

How does one deal with carboxyhemoglobinemia, anemia, and erythrocythemia? It is self-evident that these conditions will affect the amount of CO transferred from the alveolar gas to the red cells in the alveolar capillaries, but there are differences in how that effect is handled in different laboratories. Our laboratory routinely measures COHgb and estimate hemoglobin using cooximetry of venous or arterial blood if the latter is being drawn for a clinical reason. Our laboratory does not reduce predicted DLCO values in the presence of significant carboxyhemoglobin, i.e., values over 3%. Our laboratory corrects the predicted values for DLCO and DLCO/VA' for anemia and polycythemia. There are no ideal studies of the change with severe anemia, but theoretically the DLCO should be zero if there is no RBC in the pulmonary capillaries. Most studies report changes in DLCO with changes in hemoglobin from 8 to 20 g/100 mL of blood. Collected data could support either a curvilinear relationship between DLCO and anemia or a linear relationship with a Y intercept well above zero to "correct" or modify the predicted DLCO. Our laboratory uses the equations of Clark et al.[11] recommended by the ATS/ERS Task Force:[10] for men, DLCO predicted for hemoglobin (Hgb) in g/dL = DLCO predicted × (1.7 × Hgb/(10.22 + Hgb). For women, DLCO predicted for hemoglobin (Hgb) in g/dL = DLCO predicted × (1.7 × Hgb/(9.38 + Hgb).

Some laboratories do not modify the predicted value of DLCO but correct the measured value by a similar fraction. With either method, it is appropriate for the laboratory to include in their reports the following information: (1) if hemoglobin is estimated or measured; (2) if predicted DLCO is corrected for blood hemoglobin concentration, and/or (3) if measured DLCO is corrected for blood hemoglobin concentration.

Fractioning DLCO

Some investigators have factored the DLCO into components; the diffusing capacity of the alveolar membrane (Dm), the volume of blood in the pulmonary capillaries (Vc) and the reaction rate of CO with oxyhemoglobin (θ) which varies inversely with the partial pressure of O_2. The relationship between these three factors and the DLCO has been expressed as $1/DLCO = 1/Dm + 1/(θ × Vc)$ (The separation of DLCO into these factors requires measuring the DLCO at two different concentration of O_2). Further details of the necessary methodology, inferences and calculations can be found elsewhere.[10]

OTHER CONDITIONS

Hemoglobin and Obesity

We covered earlier the importance of knowing and recording the hemoglobin concentration and presence of carboxyhemoglobin or methemoglobin as they reduce measured values of DLCO. During the breath-holding period when the valve is closed preventing exhalation, Valsalva maneuvers decrease the DLCO and Mueller maneuvers increase the DLCO due to their influence on pulmonary capillary blood volume. Obesity usually increases the DLCO, especially since predicted values are usually based on age, height and gender, and not on weight. The presumed reason for slightly higher DLCO values and considerably higher DLCO/VA' values in obesity is probably the increased blood volume and the likelihood of pooling of a larger blood volume in the lung with lung size often less than mean predicted.

Aging and Heart Disease

The DLCO gradually, but very slowly, declines in apparently normal older individuals. The reasons are not clear, but they probably relate to gradual loss of capillary volume due to recognized or unrecognized illnesses, loss of capillarity and elastic recoil due to gradual destruction of alveolar walls, and unrecognized low grade heart failure. With more overt heart failure, congestion in the pulmonary veins may cause an increase in DLCO, or with pulmonary edema, a decrease in DLCO. With mitral stenosis, the DLCO is likely to be increased in earlier years, but with persistence, the vascular bed is damaged and DLCO declines. Congenital heart disease with left to right shunts, the DLCO may be increased for many years due to increased pulmonary blood flow before declining due to the development of pulmonary vascular disease. With right to left shunts, the DLCO tends to decrease.

Obstructive Lung Disease

With chronic bronchitis alone, the DLCO, VA' and DLCO/VA' are usually minimally affected or not affected but the VA'/TLC is decreased. With emphysema the DLCO is decreased while the DLCO/VA' is more severely decreased due to destruction of the alveolar walls with their capillaries. With asthma in remission, the DLCO and DLCO/VA' are often, but not always, elevated, especially in younger asthmatics. During an attack, when obstruction is severe, DLCO, DLCO/VA', VA' and VA'/TLC are all likely to be decreased.

Interstitial and Infiltrative Lung Disease

With interstitial lung disease the DLCO and VA' and usually the DLCO/VA' are decreased with minimal to moderate reduction in the VA'/TLC. In immunological lung disorders, the DLCO is often decreased even though the patient does not specifically complain about shortness of breath.

Pulmonary Vascular Disease

With chromic embolic disease, the DLCO commonly decreases. With pulmonary infarctions, the VA' and TLC also decrease. Sometimes, with a fresh lung infarction, the DLCO increases because the hemorrhagic stagnant blood in the lung quickly removes the CO from the inspired gas mixture. Pulmonary vasculopathy, which is later usually followed by pulmonary hypertension, often but not always has a reduced DLCO without any evidence of restriction or airway obstruction.

Maldistribution of Ventilation

Whenever the VA'/TLC is reduced, there are volumes of the lung to which the inspired bulk flow ventilation has not been distributed. In this situation, one should always recheck the recorded tracings and values of both the VA' and TLC measurements to see if there might be an error. If the measures are valid, one must conclude that there is maldistribution of ventilation and that consequently some volumes of the lung have not been exposed to the inspired gases. The degree of perfusion or lack of perfusion in that portion of the lung is unknown from the pulmonary function laboratory tests. But one knows that their ventilation is not optimal.

SELECTING REFERENCE VALUES

DLCO

Thirteen equations for men for DLCO were selected and analyzed at nine conditions (three heights of 165, 175, and 185 cm with ages of 30, 50, and 70 years).[12-24] These results are displayed in figure 7-3. For a 185 cm tall 30-year-old man the values ranged

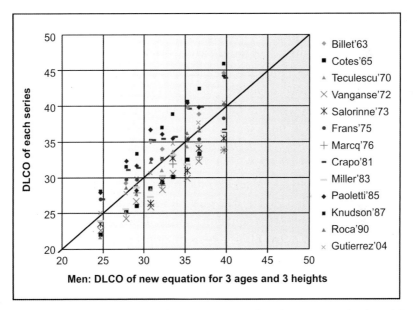

Figure 7-3 The calculated values for DLCO in mL/min/mmHg are displayed for all reference equations from 13 series of men by first authors and dates of publication given in the legend. The horizontal axis and the diagonal line of identity give the values of the newly derived equation (DLCO = −10.06 + 0.3043 × cm − 0.22 × years); the vertical axis displays the individual results of each combination of heights and ages. On the horizontal axis, they are, from left to right, 165 cm and 70 years, 175 cm and 70 years, 165 cm and 50 years, 185 cm and 70 years, 175 cm and 50 years, 165 cm and 30 years, 185 cm and 50 years, 175 cm and 30 years, and 185 cm and 30 years.

from 33.9 to 46.0 mL/min/mmHg and for a 165 cm 70-year-old man from 21.8 to 28.1 mL/min/mmHg. The mean value at 175 cm and 50 years of age was 32.2 ± 2.9 mL/min/mmHg. A new formula for men was derived, which minimized the differences between all 13 formulas at all heights and ages and exactly equaled the average of all 13 original equations. This formula in mL/min/mmHg was: –10.06 + 0.3043 × cm –0.22 × years with an SD = 2.9. *If kPa units are used, the resultant mL/min/mmHg DLCO value should be divided by 3.0.* On average, the new formula DLCO values are less than only 0.6 DLCO units away from the values of Gutierrez et al series. The mean Syx, RSD or SEE of these 13 series is 4.52. The 95% LLN values are therefore 4.52 × 1.645 = 7.42 units below the mean value of the equation for men. Thus the LLN values for tall and younger men are approximately 81% of mean predicted, for shorter older men are approximately 70% of mean predicted, and for men of median age and height 77% of mean predicted. Since the variability between series is less with lower DLCO values and higher with higher DLCO values, it is reasonable to consider the LLN as 77% of mean predicted for all ages and heights.

Nine equations for women[13-20,25] for DLCO were similarly analyzed. For a 170 cm tall 30-year-old woman the values ranged 21.9 to 31.5 mL/min/mmHg, and for a 150 cm tall 70-year-old woman the values ranged 12.1-22.2 mL/min/mmHg. The mean value at 160 cm and 50 years of age was 20.4 ± 2.61 mL/min/mmHg. A new formula for women which minimized the differences at all heights and ages for all nine original equations. This formula in mL/min/mmHg is –4.34 + 0.20944 × cm –0.139 × years with a SD of 2.9. *If kPa units are used, resultant mL/min/ mmHg DLCO value should be divided by 3.0.* On average, the new formula DLCO values are less than 0.3 DLCO units away from the values of Gutierrez et al series. The mean Syx, RSD or SEE of these nine series is 3.78. The 95% LLN values are therefore 3.78 × 1.645 = 6.22 units below the mean value of the equation for men. Thus, the LLN values for tall and younger women are approximately 81% of mean predicted; for shorter older women are approximately 63% of mean predicted, and for women of median age and height 72% of mean predicted. Thus, it is reasonable to consider the LLN as 77% of mean predicted for men and 72% for women of all ages and heights. Alternatively, and more realistic, one could consider 75% of mean predicted as the LLN for all adults (Figure 7-4).

VA' and DLCO/VA'

What Not to Do

There are some texts and manuscripts which recommended that the TLC measured by plethysmography or prolonged N_2 washout or prolonged helium dilution be used instead of the VA' measurement made during the single-breath test to determine

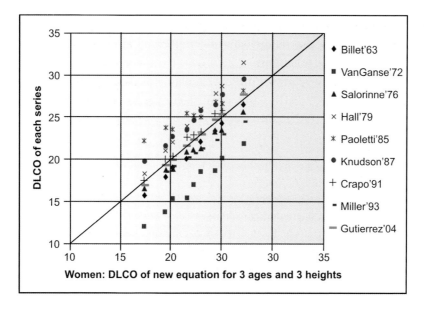

Figure 7-4 The calculated values for DLCO in mL/min/mmHg are displayed for all reference equations from nine series of women by first authors and dates of publication given in the legend. The horizontal axis and the diagonal line of identity give the values of the newly derived equation (DLCO = −4.34 + 0.20944 × cm −0.139 × years); the vertical axis displays the individual results of each combination of heights and ages. On the horizontal axis, they are, from left to right, 150 cm and 70 years, 160 cm and 70 years, 150 cm and 50 years, 170 cm and 70 years, 160 cm and 50 years, 150 cm and 30 years, 170 cm and 50 years, 160 cm and 30 years, and 170 cm and 30 years.

the maximal DLC O. They use the measured plethysmographic TLC divided by the measured single breath VA' and multiply that value by the ratio of the measured DLCO/VA'. This calculation yields a larger DLCO than that actually and validly measured. This approach is unacceptable. There is no way to know how effectively the CO might be transferred in the lung that did not receive the inert gas and CO during the 10-second maneuver.

What to Do

For predicted VA values one should select the same TLC values that are used for predicting TLC (Chapter 6). Other options are to use one or more of the following formulas: for men: predicted VA' = predicted VC/(0.8578 − 0.00333 × years of age) and for women: predicted VA' = predicted VC/(0.8385 − 0.00369 × years of age).[26] The predicted DLCO/VA' is the quotient of the predicted DLCO value in the prior section and the VA' in this section. None of the formulas for DLCO or DLCO/VA' take body weight into consideration, but it is well known that the DLCO and especially the DLCO/VA' usually rise mildly with uncomplicated moderate obesity. Use this knowledge in your interpretations.

One can also use the following direct formulas[26] for DLCO/VA'.

For men, DLCO/VA' = 9.31 − 0.018 × cm − 0.03 × years of age.

For women, DLCO/VA' = 9.58 − 0.024 × cm − 0.024 × years of age.

REFERENCES

1. Krogh A, Krogh M. Rate of diffusion of CO into the lungs of man. *Skand Arch Physiol.* 1909;23:236-47.

2. Filley GF, MacIntosh DJ, Wright GW. CO uptake and pulmonary diffusing capacity in normal subjects at rest and during exercise. *J Clin Invest.* 1954;33:530-9.

3. Riley RL, Shepard RH, Cohn JE, et al. Maximal diffusing capacity of lungs. *J Appl Physiol.* 1954;6:573-87.

4. Forster RE. Exchange of gases between alveolar air and pulmonary capillary blood: pulmonary diffusing capacity. *Physiol Rev.* 1957;37:291-452.

5. Shepard RJ. Breath-holding measurement of carbon monoxide diffusing capacity. Comparison of a field test with steady-state and other methods of measurement. *J Physiol (London).* 1958;141:408-18.

6. Ogilvie CM, Forster RE, Blakemore WS, et al. A standardized breath holding technique for the clinical measurement of the diffusing capacity of the lung for carbon monoxide. *J Clin Invest.* 1957;36:1-17.

7. Burrows B, Kasik JE, Niden AH, et al. Clinical usefulness of the single-breath pulmonary diffusing capacity test. *Am Rev Respir Dis.* 1961;84:789-806.

8. Jones RS, Meade F. A theoretical and experimental analysis of anomalies in the estimation of pulmonary diffusing capacity by the single-breath method. *Q J Exp Physiol Cogn Med Sci.* 1961;46:131-43.

9. Ferris BG. Epidemiolog Standardization Project (American Thoracic Society). *Am Rev Respir Dis.* 1978;118:1-120.

10. MacIntyre N, Crapo RO, Viegi DC, et al. ATS/ERS task force: standardisation of the single-breath determination of carbon monoxide uptake in the lung. *Eur Respir J.* 2005;26:720-35.

11. Clark EH, Woods RL, Hughes JMB. Effect of blood transfusion on the carbon monoxide transfer factor of the lung in man. *Clin Sci.* 1972;42:325-35.

12. Cotes JE. Lung Function: Assessment and Application in Medicine, 4th edition. Oxford: Blackwell Scientific Publications; 1979.

13. Billiet L, Baisier W, Naedts JP. Effet de la taille, et du sefe de l'age sur la capacitie de diffusion pulmonaire de l'adult normal. *J Physiol (Paris).* 1963;55:199-200.

14. VanGanse WF, Ferris BJ Jr, Cotes JE. Cigarette smoking and pulmonary diffusing capacity (transfer factor). *Am Rev Respir Dis.* 1972;105:30-41.

15. Salorinne Y. Single-breath pulmonary diffusing capacity: reference values and application in connective tissue diseases and in various lung diseases. *Scand J Respir Dis.* 1976;96 (Suppl):1-86.

16. Crapo RO, Morris AH. Standardized single-breath normal values for diffusing capacity. *Am Rev Respir Dis*. 1981;123:185-9.

17. Miller A, Thornton JC, Warshaw R, et al. Single breath diffusing capacity in a representative sample of the population of Michigan, a large industrial state. Predicted values, lower limits of normal, and frequencies of abnormality by smoking history. *Am Rev Respir Dis*. 1983;127:270-7.

18. Paoletti P, Viegi G, Pistellio G, et al. Reference equations for the single-breath diffusing capacity. A cross-sectional analysis and effect of body size and age. *Am Rev Respir Dis*. 1985;132:806-13.

19. Knudson RJ, Kaltenborn WT, Knudson DE, et al. The single-breath carbon monoxide diffusing capacity. Reference equations derived from a healthy nonsmoking population and effects of hematocrit. *Am Rev Respir Dis*. 1987;135:805-11.

20. Gutierrez C, Ghezzo RH, Abboud RT, et al. Reference values of pulmonary function tests for Canadian Caucasians. *Can Respir J*. 2004;11:414-24.

21. Teculescu DB, Stanescu DC. Lung diffusing capacity. Normal values in male smokers and non-smokers using the breath-holding technique. *Scand J Respir Dis*. 1970;51:137-49.

22. Frans A, Stanescu DC, Veriter C, et al. Smoking and pulmonary diffusing capacity. *Scand J Respir Dis*. 1975;56:165-83.

23. Marcq M, Minette A. Lung function changes in smokers with normal conventional spirometry. *Am Rev Respir Dis*. 1976;114:723-38.

24. Roca J, Rodriquez-Roisin R, Cobo E, et al. Single-breath carbon monoxide diffusing capacity prediction equations from a Mediterranean population. *Am Rev Respir Dis*. 1990;141:1026-32.

25. Hall AM, Heywood C, Cotes JE. Lung function in healthy British women. *Thorax*. 1979;34:359-65.

26. Hansen JE. Unpublished observations.

8 Single Breath O₂ Test

HISTORY AND THEORY OF MEASUREMENT

It has been known for many years that inhaled gases were not equally distributed to all portions of the lung. This differential distribution was in part dependent on gravity, since the superior and inferior alveoli were approximately equal in size at full inspiration, but after full exhalation the superior airspaces were considerably larger than those at the bases. Thus, the airspace sizes did not change equally at the lung apex and lung bases during large tidal volume breathing so that inhaled gases were not equally distributed throughout the lung. This is fortunate, because blood flow is also gravity dependent and is not equally distributed throughout the lung. In the early 1950s attempts were made to assess the distribution of inhaled gases by injecting boluses of an insoluble foreign gas into the inspired gases and measuring its concentrations during exhalation.[1]

In 1970, Anthonisen et al. modified this approach by monitoring only the dominant resident gas in the lung (N_2). The procedure required inhaling a vital capacity-sized quantity of 100% O_2 and evaluating the evenness of the exhalation of N_2 during the subsequent exhalation.[2] On a graph one could compare the volume exhaled on the X-axis with the concentration of N_2 on the Y-axis. This allowed several factors to be evaluated: (1) The volume of the initial exhaled gas that was without N_2, (2) the volume exhaled before the N_2 concentration was relatively stable, (3) the volume and stability of the concentration of N_2 during the major portion of the exhalation, and (4) the frequent increase in N_2 concentration near the end of the forced exhalation.[3]

These consecutive four phases became identified as phases 1, 2, 3, and 4. Phase 1 washed out the O_2 in the mouth and largest airways; Phase 2 continued the washout of O_2 from the smaller airways; Phase 3, or the alveolar plateau, was evidence of the distribution of O_2 to the majority of airspaces; while the Phase 4 volume, also identified as the closing volume (CV), was evidence of the distribution of O_2 to the remainder of the airspaces as the lung was compressed to its smallest volume. In a normal individual, the small but gradual increase in N_2 concentration during phase 3, the alveolar plateau, was evidence of the relatively even distribution of the O_2 to the majority of the airspaces (Figure 8-1).

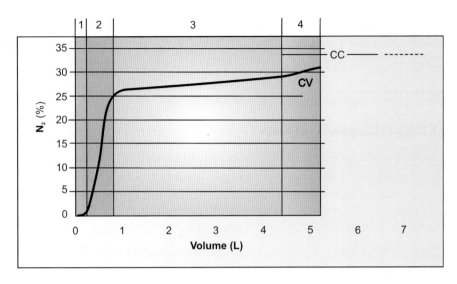

Figure 8-1 Display of a normal single breath O_2 test. Exhaled volume is on the X-axis and % N_2 is on the Y-axis. After an inhalation of 100% O_2, the subject slowly exhales the vital capacity; in this case, it is about 5 L. CC = closing capacity; CV = closing volume. The four phases are labeled 1, 2, 3 and 4. Phase 1 (green) is considered large airway dead space. Phase 2 (blue) is the abrupt rise to Phase 3 (magenta) the alveolar plateau. Phase 4 (orange) is the closing volume. The closing capacity, which is the closing volume plus the residual volume cannot be measured without knowing the total lung capacity.

In the 1970s, because of the realization of the devastating health effects of cigarette smoking, there were many attempts to find methodology to better objectively quantify evidence of airway damage from smoking. This led to the development of reference values for both closing volumes (phase 4) and the slope of phase 3 in never-smoking adults for comparisons with the values found in smokers.[4,5] Although measurements of phase 3 values as then defined and phase 4 values to detect early or small airways disease were not widely clinically adopted, the changes seen in the tracings are revealing and can be useful in identifying maldistribution of ventilation.

In individuals with airway obstruction it is logical to expect that the alveolar plateau will be steeper than in individuals without airway obstruction. The plateau is also steeper in lungs that have volumes with differing compliances due to patches of fibrosis or emphysema.

The closing volume is attributable to airway closure at the bases of the lungs near the end of exhalation (See Figure 2-21 in Chapter 2). In the upright position, from complete exhalation to complete inhalation (RV to TLC), the airspace sizes at the bases change more than those at the apices. Consequently the lung base airspaces, after the inhalation of 100% O_2, have a larger concentration of O_2 and lower concentration of N_2 than those at the lung apices. When, during late exhalation, the basilar airspaces are "closed off", the remaining exhaled volume has a lower concentration of O_2 and a higher concentration of N_2.

MAKING THE MEASUREMENT

The subject is seated quietly with a nose clip and mouthpiece. After the subject exhales completely to RV, a valve is turned into a bag or spirometer with 100% O_2, from which the subject rapidly inhales a full VC to TLC. Immediately the valve is turned allowing the subject to exhale slowly to RV. Meanwhile, on an X-Y recorder, the N_2 concentration at the mouth is recorded on the Y-axis while the volume of exhalation is recorded on the X-axis. After a short wait, the measure can be repeated. In subjects with normal or moderate disease, the phases can be clearly differentiated manually on the tracing. Interestingly, some commercial systems do not use a N_2 meter. Instead, they use O_2 and CO_2 analyzers to calculate and display %N_2 changes.

CALCULATIONS

With the assistance of a transparent ruler, a line can be drawn through phase 3 showing slope of the alveolar plateau. A vertical arrow or line can be placed where phase 3 changes to phase 4. The slope of the line has traditionally been measured as a percent change of N_2/L of volume. The closing volume (CV or phase 4) is expressed as a percent of total VC. On occasion a change in slope cannot be identified separating phase 4 from phase 3. In most commercial systems, software is used to calculate and report the difference between the N_2 concentration at 750 mL and 1250 mL as a slope value.

The slope of phase 3 has traditionally been measured manually or by computer software as a change of percent N_2/L over the 500 mL volume, i.e., from 750 mL to 1250 mL. There are several reasons why using software may not be optimal: (1) In individuals with a large VC, the alveolar plateau (phase 3) does not begin until after 750 mL of exhalation, a point of exhalation which is still on the "knee" before phase 2 changes to phase 3. (2) In individuals with small VC, the alveolar plateau (phase 3) may be ended before 1250 mL has been exhaled and phase 4 has begun. (3) Oscillations in some tracings, due to cardiac pulsations, give inordinately high or low slope values because one or both of the 750 mL and 1250 mL values happen to be at the top or bottom of the oscillations. Thus, connecting the exact 750 mL and 1250 mL points may give falsely lower or higher slopes. Additional objections will soon be discussed.

NORMAL VALUES

Comroe, Forster, and colleagues,[6] in their second edition of "The Lung", have somewhat conflicting suggestions, but always uses the percent increase over 500 mL rather than percent increase per liter. An increase of 1.5% over 500 mL is the same as a 3.0% increase per liter. In 26 normal subjects under age 50, they found that the %N$_2$ increase from 750–1250 mL never exceeded 1.5%. In 25 normal subjects over age 50, the %N$_2$ increase was 1.8% ± 1.1% with a maximum of 4.5% for 500 mL. In patients with asthma, emphysema, bronchiectasis, sarcoid, congestive heart failure, pulmonary carcinoma, and post-pneumonectomy, mean increases were 3.0–6.9% N$_2$ per 500 mL.

It is stated in the appendix of "The Lung" that the %N$_2$ increase for 500 mL of expired alveolar air should be less than 1.5%, with no age, gender, or height condition. Some of their specific single breath values are reported in table 8-1. Buist and Ross present their recommendations for upper limits of normal for the change in %N$_2$ per liter for 750–1250 mL in table 8-2.

In both series, the percent change allowed increases with age, but normal values can be considerably higher for Comroe et al.[6] than for Buist and Ross.[5]

Table 8-1	Single Breath O$_2$ Values as Reported and Evaluated by Comroe et al.[6] in the Lung, by size of VC and Subject Age				
VC (L)	Case #	Age, (years)	% change from 750 to 1250 (mL)	% change per L	Called Normal (N) or Abnormal (A)
1.3	8	28	7	14	A
1.5	9	45	2	4	N
1.6	8	25	3	6	A
1.7	5	63	3	6	A
1.9	8	22	2	4	N
2.8	3	17	3	6	A
3.4	6	39	7.4	14.8	A
4.1	6	39	2.7	5.4	N
4.2	10	38	4	8	A
4.3	1	63	1.3	2.6	N
4.6	12	38	4	8	A
5.9	13	18	1.5	3	N

Table 8-2	Single Breath O_2 Values Upper Limit of Normal as Reported and Evaluated by Buist and Ross[5]	
Age (years)	Men, % increase N_2 per L	Women, % increase N_2 per L
20	1.6	2.2
30	1.7	2.2
40	1.8	2.3
50	1.9	2.4
60	2.0	2.5
65	2.1	3.8
70	2.1	4.4
80	2.2	5.0

INTERPRETATIONS

It is usually easy and painless to obtain single breath O_2 tests. Rather than over-interpreting the numbers, it is clear that looking at the curves gives one a "gestalt" or impression as to whether or not there is significant maldistribution of ventilation. During asthma attacks, for example, the overall rises in N_2 are steep throughout the exhalation so that distinction between phases 1 and 2 or 2 and 3 is difficult. In such a case, there is certainly severe maldistribution of ventilation.

Closing volumes are also affected by obesity independent of the presence or absence of intrinsic lung disease, due to the likelihood of increased basilar atelectasis near RV in obese individuals. Closing capacities, which are determined by adding the CV to the RV measured by other techniques, seems to offer no advantages over the measurement of RV or RV/TLC measured by N_2 washout, helium dilution, or plethysmography to ascertain if there is air-trapping or hyperinflation.

Please consider why using the same standard of normalcy for the change in $\%N_2$/L is inappropriate. Consider the situation of two apparently normal individuals who differ markedly in size. The larger subject has a VC of 6.0 L and the smaller subject has a VC of 2.0 L. Their SBO_2 tracings are given in figure 8-2.

RECOMMENDATIONS

It may be better to report an overall impression of the tracing rather than relying exclusively on absolute slope values. If a laboratory reports previously published reference and actual measured values of the single breath O_2 test in ΔN_2/L in all individuals including one with a small VC, the recipient of the report may be puzzled

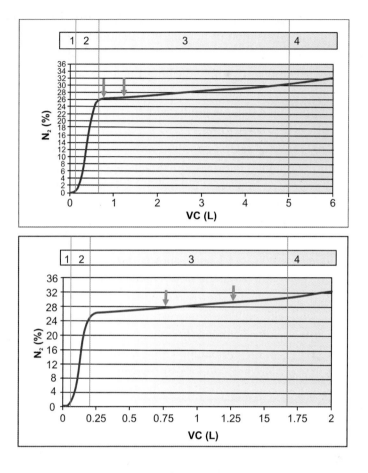

Figure 8-2 Figure showing why measuring slope from 750-1250 mL is poor. It also shows single breath O$_2$ tracings of two normal individuals. Exhaled volumes are on both X-axes; percent N$_2$ are on both Y-axes. Phases 1, 2, 3, and 4 are separated by vertical lines. The subject in the upper tracing has a VC of 6.0 L while the subject in the lower tracing has a VC of 2.0 L. The 750-1250 mL slopes are identified in both tracings. Note that the pattern and absolute values of %N$_2$ over the full tracings from complete inhalation to complete exhalation are identical. In the upper tracing the %ΔN$_2$ is 0.5% from 750-1250 mL, which is equal to 1.0% N$_2$/L. In the lower tracing the %ΔN$_2$ is 1.5% from 750-1250 mL is equal to 3.0% N$_2$/L. It is illogical to judge the individual with the VC of 2.0 L as having an abnormal single breath O$_2$ test while the individual with a VC of 6.0 L has a normal single breath O$_2$. This illustrates the fallacy in interpreting single breath oxygen tests by using %ΔN$_2$ per 500 mL or %ΔN$_2$/L as a standard.

by a higher actual value than the predicted value printed few centimeters away on the report and the interpretation of normalcy. The finding of a high $\Delta N_2/L$ in an individual with restrictive lung disease may be due to maldistribution of ventilation due to differences in compliance within the lung, but it may also be due to the use of Liters in the denominator rather than a fraction of the measured VC. It is appropriate to state in the interpretation that the predicted $\Delta N_2/L$ value may be of questionable validity in individuals with small lungs.

The historically-reported reference values of $\%\Delta N_2/L$ are not optimal because they do not well differentiate between individuals of differing sizes. Thus, values for the slope are expressed in percent change in N_2/L, regardless of the volume of the VC. Because of difference in individual sizes and their VC's, the percent change could have been more properly expressed as percent change per a given fraction of the VC. For example, in two normal individuals of the same age but differing sizes, a taller person might have a VC of 6 L and a shorter person a VC of 2 L. If the $\%\Delta N_2/L$ were 3.0%/L in the taller individual the slope change would be 3% for 1/6 of the VC. If the $\%\Delta N_2/L$ were 3.0%/L in the shorter individual, the slope change would be 3% for 1/2 of the VC. Thus, although the slopes expressed as $\%\Delta N_2/L$ are similar in both individuals, it clearly rises three times as fast per total VC in the taller individual. Yet, using published standards for normal individuals, one would be forced to use the same standards to ascertain if the slopes were within normal limits or further than 1.65 or 2.0 SD away from mean predicted $\Delta N_2/L$. Thus, the individual with a smaller VC, whether due to age, gender, disease, or height, with the same slope calculated in $\Delta N_2/L$, will be considered more abnormal by $\Delta N_2/L$ than an individual with a larger VC if historical values are used.

Therefore, considering the previously reported values and discussion it is suggested that the approximate upper limit of normal for change in $\%N_2$ in the alveolar plateau (phase 3) should be as shown in figure 8-3, i.e., 2.0% for one-quarter of the VC, regardless of age or gender. Thus for a VC of 2 L, upper limit of normal (ULN) for $\%\Delta N_2/L$ would be 4.0%, for a VC of 4 L, ULN for $\%\Delta N_2/L$ would be 2.0%, for a VC of 6 L, ULN for $\%\Delta N_2/L$ would be 1.33%. Thus, the ULN value can also be calculated in $\%\Delta N_2/L$ by dividing 8.0 by the VC in L.

In conclusion, the problem of defining normalcy can be solved by using the normal values recommended in figure 8-3 to interpret the single breath O_2 test.[7] As noted in chapter 7, maldistribution of ventilation can also be assessed by using the VA'/TLC ratio. With a valid DLCO and VA' test, a VA'/TLC of less than 80 to 90%, both measured, indicates significant maldistribution of ventilation. Maldistribution measured by a single breath O_2 test usually correlates reasonably well with maldistribution measured by the VA'/TLC ratio.[7]

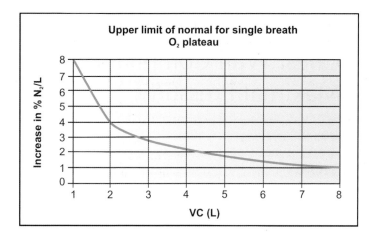

Figure 8-3 Recommended upper limit of normal for the %ΔN₂/L of the alveolar plateau, phase 3. Neither phase 2 or phase 4 should be included. The slope should be determined by ignoring undulations. The normal value when expressed in %ΔN₂ is dependent on the VC. The upper limit value can also be calculated by dividing the number 8 by the VC in Liters.

REFERENCES

1. Fowler WS. Lung function studies; uneven pulmonary ventilation in normal subjects and in patients with pulmonary disease. *J Appl Physiol*. 1949; 2(6):283-99.
2. Anthonisen NR, Danson J, Robertson PC, et al. Airway closure as a function of age. *Respir Physiol*. 1969; 8(1):58-65.
3. Buist AS, Van Fleet DL, Ross BB. A comparison of conventional spirometric tests and the test of closing volume in an emphysema screening center. *Am Rev Respir Dis*. 1973; 107(5):735-43.
4. Buist AS. Early detection of airways obstruction by the closing volume technique. *Chest*. 1973; 64(4):495-9.
5. Buist AS, Ross BB. Quantitative analysis of the alveolar plateau in the diagnosis of early airway obstruction. *Am Rev Respir Dis*. 1973; 108(5):1078-87.
6. Comreo JH Jr, Forster RE II, DuBois AB, Briscoe WA, Corlsen E. The lung: Clinical Physiology and Pulmonary function tesats (2nd edn). Chicago: Yearbook, 1982;390.
7. Hansen JE. Unpublished observations.

CHAPTER 9 Airway Resistance, Lung and Chest Wall Compliance and Maximal Pressures

INTRODUCTION

Measurements of airway resistance and lung and chest wall compliance are of interest in understanding the normal physiology and pathophysiology of ventilation. These tests are used in some research studies but are of limited value in patient care. Airway resistance is measured during plethysmography. Compliance measurements require insertion of an esophageal balloon or catheter to reflect intrapleural pressure changes during carefully performed ventilatory maneuvers. Readers are referred to listed references for details of making and interpreting these measurements.[1]

Maximal inspiratory pressure (MIP) and maximal expiratory pressure (MEP) measurements are not routinely performed in the clinical laboratory, but are non-invasive, relatively simple, easy to understand, and sometimes clinically useful. They primarily measure ventilatory muscle strength and are dependent on the lung volume at which measured. Generally, these pressures decrease with neuromuscular disease and age. They are higher in men than women, and can sometimes be improved with training and exercise.

EQUIPMENT AND PERFORMANCE OF MAXIMAL PRESSURE TESTS

The pressure measuring device for both maximal pressure tests consists of a mouthpiece with a rubber, plastic, paper, or metal flange, connected through a filter to a plastic or metal tube of the approximate same diameter as the mouthpiece. The tube is usually closed at the distal end, sometimes by a three-way valve. If there is no valve at the end, there is an opening in the side of the tube, perhaps a centimeter in diameter, which can be occluded by a finger to obstruct flow when pressures are measured. The tube also has a small opening, perhaps 1-2 mm in diameter, which serves as a leak and also a connection to a pressure-measuring device. The pressure measuring device may be a transducer or manometer which can be calibrated against a column of mercury. The location of these two holes does not appear to be critical. Devices for clinical testing, including manometers or transducers, are commercially available.

During the test, the patient is seated comfortably with the nostrils occluded. For maximal inspiratory pressures (MIP), the measurements are made as close as possible to RV. For maximal expiratory pressures (MEP), the measurements are made as close as possible to TLC. Pressure measurements made in the tidal volume or FRC range are considerably less than those near RV or TLC. The patient is instructed to hold maximal inspiratory or expiratory efforts for about three seconds. Both the peak value and the average value during a one-second period can be recorded. The highest one-second average is ordinarily the one finally reported. MIP tests are usually performed before MEP tests. A maximal number of 3 to 5 MIP and 3 to 5 MEP tests are suggested with a rest period of one minute between each test. When efforts appear to be maximal and the highest one-second average values are within 10-15% of each other, testing is completed and considered to be valid.

NORMAL VALUES AND INTERPRETATION OF MAXIMAL PRESSURE TESTS

Because of the high variability of the tests in an individual even at one sitting and the apparent dependence on operator skills, 95% confidence limits lower limit of normal (LLN) pressure values are more clinically important than mean pressure values. A recent review article[2] suggests the following reference equations for adults up to age 70 years, reporting pressures in cm H_2O (13.7 cm of water = 10 mmHg):

Men mean MIP = 120 – (0.41 × age in years); LLN MIP = 62 – (0.15 × age in years)

Men mean MEP = 174 – (0.83 × age in years); LLN MEP = 117 – (0.83 × age in years)

Women mean MIP = 108 – (0.61 × age in years); LLN MIP = 62 – (0.50 × age in years)

Women mean MEP = 131 – (0.86 × age in years); LLN MEP = 95 – (0.57 × age in years)

A multiethnic study of MIP but not MEP[3] was recently published in the same issue of the same journal reporting mean and LLN values in over 3000 relatively healthy adults between the ages of 45 and 84 years. The subjects were part of an atherosclerosis study. The authors noted no significant ethnic/race differences, but did note higher MIP values in men and younger subjects and those with obesity, higher FVC and shorter heights. Their LLN values agree reasonably well (within 10 cm of H_2O) with those of Evans and Whitelaw for men of average size between the ages of 65–75 but not at other ages. They are 10–20 cm of water higher for women of average size from ages 50–80 years.

Thus, it appears reasonable to conclude that there is considerable variability between mean and LLN values from different studies, in part related to differences in equipment and techniques. Therefore, unless maximal pressure values are quite low, results of a single test should be cautiously interpreted. Serial tests in the same individual in the same laboratory are likely to be of more clinical value.

REFERENCES

1. American Thoracic Society/European Respiratory Society. ATS/ERS statement on respiratory muscle testing. *Am J Respir Crit Care Med.* 2002; 166(4):518-624.

2. Evans JA, Whitelaw WA. The assessment of maximal respiratory mouth pressures in adults. *Respir Care.* 2009; 54(10):1348-59.

3. Sachs MC, Enright PL, Hinckley Stukovsky KD, et al. Performance of maximal inspiratory pressure tests and maximum inspiratory pressure reference equations for 4 race/ethnic groups. *Respir Care.* 2009; 54(10):1321-8.

10 Blood Gases and pH

BACKGROUND

There are individuals who would say that a chapter on blood gases and pH properly belongs in a book emphasizing nephrology, anesthesiology, intensive care medicine, exercise physiology, cardiology, surgery, general internal medicine, emergency medicine, obstetrics, sports medicine, military medicine, or epidemiology..., and each would be correct. They might site the roles of Van Slyke, Henderson, Hasselbalch, Barcroft, Haldane, Dill, Cournand, Scholander, Astrup, Riley, Davenport, Clark, Rahn, Severinghaus, or West..., and they would be correct. We are grateful for their contributions and those of their collaborators and others not named here.

We will consider measurements within or outside of the pulmonary function laboratory of arterial, mixed venous and capillary blood specimens, although other fluid specimens can also be analyzed. Present day equipment routinely measures pH, [H+], pCO_2, pO_2, and oxyhemoglobin saturation, with calculations of $[HCO_3^-]$, base excess and SaO_2. In some equipment, additional measures of carboxyhemoglobin, methemoglobin, glucose, lactate, chloride, sodium, calcium, and potassium can be made. In this chapter we will consider only measurements and interpretations of acid-base status and oxygenation in blood specimens.

PRE-ANALYSIS FACTORS: PATIENTS, SPECIMEN IDENTIFICATION, TIMING, COLLECTION AND TRANSPORT

The patient may not always be stable when the blood specimen is obtained but it is mandatory to identify the specimen with the patient's name, identification number, and time and anatomic site of collection. The specimen may be from an arterial puncture, an arterial catheter, an intracardiac or pulmonary artery catheter, a free-flowing capillary sample, or (intentionally or otherwise) even peripheral venous blood. If there are bubbles in the specimen, they should be immediately removed. The specimen should be obtained in a heparinized capillary tube or a small syringe, preferably heparin coating or tablets rather than liquid heparin, since liquid heparin dilutes (reduces) CO_2 values and may raise O_2 values.[1]

If the specimen is being measured on-site, that is with point of care analysis, it should not be iced. Despite the common custom of icing blood specimens, this is not necessary or wise when the specimen is promptly analyzed.[2] An exception might be made and icing reasonable if the blood specimen contains over 20,000 white blood cells, as metabolism by these cells can reduce pO_2 slightly and increase pCO_2, [H^+] and lactate. The reasons for not-icing are as follows: Icing a specimen is messy, consumes resources, and may delay transport of the specimen. When blood is collected in plastic syringes, especially if the sample is small in proportion to the syringe size, O_2 diffuses into the specimen from the ice water surrounding the syringe barrel and CO_2 can diffuse out. The latter is of minor consequence, but if the blood pO_2 is on the upper or flat part of the oxyhemoglobin dissociation curve, the increase in pO_2 in the specimen may be significant. The dominant concern should be to transport the specimen to the blood gas laboratory so that the analysis occurs in less than 20 minutes after the specimen has been drawn from the patient.[3]

BLOOD GAS LABORATORY ANALYSIS

Equipment and Personnel

Several manufacturers have developed excellent measuring equipment for analyzing sealed blood specimens, i.e., which have not been exposed to room air. Traditionally, equipment in the pulmonary laboratory primarily measured pO_2, pCO_2, and pH.[4] Soon thereafter, co-oximetry allowed synchronous measurement of oxyhemoglobin, carboxyhemoglobin, methemoglobin, and reduced hemoglobin.[5] Now, less commonly, some pulmonary function laboratories also measure lactate, glucose, sodium, potassium, calcium, and/or chloride. Manufacturers are specific in their guidance as to how their machines should be treated and maintained. Pulmonary laboratories usually have some personnel dedicated full or part time to blood measuring equipment maintenance, quality control, proficiency testing and record maintenance.

Calibrations, Quality Control, Proficiency Testing of Equipment, and Personnel, and Analysis

For the quality of patient care and in order to obtain and maintain the approval of licensing agencies it is necessary to follow rigid rules regarding the frequency and timing of machine calibrations with known gases or liquids. Quality control liquids of specific lot numbers are obtained in individual sealed ampoules by the manufacturer. They are manufactured under strict supervision so that ampoules from the same lot number contain material which will give highly reproducible results in properly functioning equipment.[6] Because of the differences in equipment design, the target values for ampoules from a given lot often differ from model to model, even from the same manufacturer, but they should be highly reproducible in equipment of the same model.[7] Target values for one level might be $pO_2 = 80$ mmHg, $pCO_2 = 36$ mmHg, and pH = 7.42; for a second level $pO_2 = 58$ mmHg, $pCO_2 = 54$ mmHg, and pH = 7.22; and for a third level $pO_2 = 120$ mmHg, $pCO_2 = 25$ mmHg, and pH = 7.58 for a specific model. Additional ampoules at a high pO_2 level are also available for use just before testing blood from patients on O_2 suspected of having with very high pO_2 levels. For proficiency testing, ampoules are sent as unknowns to multiple laboratories for analysis, reporting, and grading.[8] The frequency of calibrations, quality control measurements, and proficiency testing measurements are set by the manufacturers, licensing agencies, and professional societies or organizations administering the proficiency testing program.

It is worth emphasizing that quality control is dependent not only on the equipment but also on the personnel using the equipment. Blood samples require meticulous recording in the laboratory (electronically or by hand) of the patient name, identification number, site, and time of collection, and proper handling of the sample within the laboratory.[3]

Making the Measurements

If the sample is in a syringe and a gas bubble is noted, that should be immediately removed. After removal of any bubble, the syringe sample should also be manipulated by hand to obtain a well-mixed specimen, or the measured hemoglobin value may not be representative. As required by the equipment, the specimen is introduced into the portal of the machine anerobically either by aspiration or pushing on the syringe barrel. The results are presented usually within a minute or so. If the results are out of range of reasonable values, it is wise to introduce a sample from the same syringe again. In some cases, the samples need to be introduced into two machines, one for pO_2 pCO_2, and pH, and the other for co-oximetry. When this is the case, the blood gas analyzer should be used first.

Reporting Results: Telephone, Computer, Slips of Paper

It is preferable to have as few steps as possible between the blood sample and those caring for the patient. Each verbal or written transmission increases the possibility of a misunderstanding or transcription error. When the results are transmitted electronically from the analyzer to the professional who obtained the blood and requested the analyses, the likelihood of error decreases. Thus it may be best to reduce these steps as much as possible and imprint or insert the laboratory results as directly as possible in the patient's medical chart or record.

POINT-OF-CARE ANALYSIS

Equipment and Personnel

Equipment is now available for performing these analyses immediately in intensive care units, emergency rooms, surgical suites, in the wards and in the clinics. The equipment is small, usually can be hand-held, and often operated by batteries so that it is fully mobile. Depending on the cartridges inserted, it can measure blood gases and pH and/or all of the electrolytes listed in Blood Gas Laboratory Analysis: Equipment and personnel. The operating personnel need not be extensively trained. In many situations the equipment is operated by nursing personnel who may have many other responsibilities.

Calibrations and Quality Control

The equipment is programmed to require calibrations in a timely manner before insertion of blood specimens.

Reporting and Recording Results

The results of point of care equipment may be displayed on a screen and written down or sent to an accessory printer. In any case, the results must be tightly identified to the patient, site and time of sampling to avert misinformation. As in receiving data from a laboratory a distance away, it is important to reduce copying and transmission errors.

INTERPRETING ACID-BASE STATUS

Terminology, pH and [H+] and Henderson-Hasselbalch Equation

Terminology is considered important. [H+] values or most commonly converted to pH values, which are the negative logarithm to the base 10 of the [H+] concentration or pressure.[9] Thus a [H+] concentration of 10^{-7} moles = pH of 7.0 is found in neutral water at 25° C; a [H+] concentration of 10^0 moles = pH of 1.0 is found in a concentrated solution of hydrochloric acid in water; and a [H+] concentration of 10^{-14} = pH of 14 is found in a concentration solution of sodium hydroxide. In the arterial blood of a normal resting human at 37° C, the usual [H+] concentration of $10^{-7.4}$ = pH of 7.4.[10] The approximate equivalent H+ concentrations paired with pH values are shown later in figure 10-3.

Because the major buffering system in the body is based on pCO_2 and [HCO_3^-] with a acid dissociation constant (pK') approximating 6.1, it is essential to use their relationships in evaluating deviations in pH or [H+] from arterial blood neutrality of pH 7.40. The Henderson-Hasselbalch equation is as follows:

$$pH = pK' + \log_{10} \frac{([HCO_3^-])}{(pCO_2 \times 0.0307)}$$

where $[HCO_3^-]$ is given in mEq/L and pCO_2 is given in mmHg or torr.[11] The pK' shifts slightly as pH changes, so that the pK' at pH 7.20 = 6.094; at pH 7.40 = 6.086; and at pH 7.60 = 6.078.[12]

First, it is important to discard the concepts shown in figure 10-1, which are almost universally displayed in textbooks to portray the relationship between pCO_2 and $[HCO_3^-]$ or pCO_2 and blood CO_2 content. This relationship is shown as curvilinear without any display of pH or $[H^+]$ concentration. If we return to the Henderson-Hasselbalch equation, it is quite clear that for any given pH or $[H^+]$ concentration, the relationship between pCO_2 and $[HCO_3^-]$ is linear. Thus, any diagram which shows

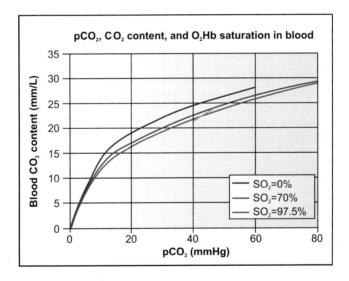

Figure 10-1 It shows the traditional graphical relationship between pCO_2 and CO_2 content in blood found in many textbooks. It does not show pH values. It purports to show the differences in CO_2 content for any given pCO_2 and oxyhemoglobin saturations (SO_2) of 0%, 70% and 97.5%. The thick blue line ascribes the difference between mixed venous and arterial pCO_2 and CO_2 contents at rest as primarily due to the Haldane effect, i.e., the difference in oxyhemoglobin saturations. As discussed in the text, this figure is very misleading on several accounts: (1) it shows a curvilinear relationship between pCO_2 and total CO_2 which is not true when pH is stable; (2) it ignores pH; (3) it incorrectly ascribes the differences between pCO_2 and total CO_2 of mixed venous and arterial blood as predominantly due to differences in oxyhemoglobin saturation. The correct relationships are shown in figures 10-2 and 10-3.

this curvilinearity includes unportrayed pH changes. Furthermore, these diagrams imply that differences between mixed venous and arterial blood oxyhemoglobin saturation are the key factor in the Haldane effect. This is incorrect, since the major cause of the difference between mixed venous and arterial CO_2 content is the pH difference between the mixed venous and arterial blood, not the difference in oxyhemoglobin saturation or O_2 content.

The figure 10-2 displays the correct relationship between blood pCO_2 and the total blood CO_2 content using appropriate pK' values for each pH value. For a given pCO_2, note the very large differences in CO_2 content due to differing pH values and the trivial differences due to oxyhemoglobin saturations of 95% and 20%. Both Y-axes of the two figures present blood CO_2 content in mM/L.

In normal humans and during disease states, the body attempts to maintain arterial pH within a narrow range, 7.40 ± 0.02. *Acidemia* is present if the pH is 7.37 or below while *alkalemia* is present when the pH is 7.43 or above. The processes which modify the acid-base status are identified as *acidosis* or *alkalosis*. If the process is

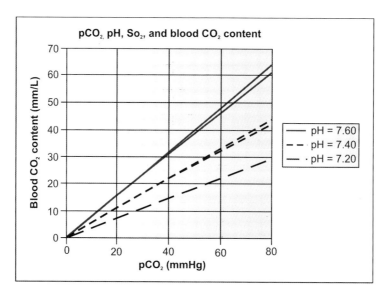

Figure 10-2 The correct relationship of pCO_2 and total blood CO_2 content. The hemoglobin is 15.0 g/dL. There are three pairs of lines; in each case the saturations of oxyhemoglobin are 20% in the upper lines and 95% in the lower lines of each pair. The three pairs of diagonal lines identify pH values of 7.60 (red), 7.40 (dotted blue) and pH 7.20 (dashed black). Note the minimal effect of oxyhemoglobin saturation on CO_2 content of whole blood (the difference between the 20% and 95% saturation lines at each pH), especially at a pH of 7.20. Note also the major dependence of CO_2 content on pCO_2 (X-axis) and pH (red, blue and black diagonal lines).

primarily the result of acute hyperventilation or hypoventilation, the processes are, respectively, acute *respiratory alkalosis* and acute *respiratory acidosis* and are represented as horizontal moves to the right or left in figure 10-3. If the respiratory process continues, the normal (and usually diseased) body attempts to bring the pH back towards 7.40 by compensatory mechanisms, i.e., decreasing the HCO_3^- for respiratory alkalosis and increasing the $[HCO_3^-]$ for respiratory acidosis. These processes are compensatory and should not be identified as primary.

If the processes, which modify the acid-base status are not respiratory, they are correctly identified as *non-respiratory acidosis* and *non-respiratory alkalosis*, but are usually more briefly identified as *metabolic acidosis* and *metabolic alkalosis*. Referring to figure 10-3,[13-17] these acute processes move vertically, with reductions in $[HCO_3^-]$ with metabolic acidosis (movement downward) and increases in $[HCO_3^-]$ with metabolic alkalosis (movement upward). With primary metabolic acidosis, the brain's respiratory center is stimulated and hyperventilation results with compensatory decline in pCO_2 and return of the pH towards 7.40. With primary metabolic alkalosis, hypoventilation normally follows with resultant increase in pCO_2. These changes in pCO_2 which follow changes in $[HCO_3^-]$ should be identified as compensatory and not as primary.

Several examples of simple disorders are given in table 10-1 using approximate numbers and calculations.[13-17] Note that it is not absolute values but the ratios of $[HCO_3^-]$ to pCO_2 that determine whether there is acidemia or alkalemia or whether the process is primarily respiratory or non-respiratory acidosis or alkalosis.

So far we have identified primary disorders and their compensations. The shaded colored areas in the diagram indicate the common $[HCO_3^-]$, pCO_2, and pH changes caused by single primary disorders including their usual compensations. It is, of course, possible for patients to have more than one primary disorder. In fact two or three or even four primary disorders are possible in a single patient. Figure 10-3 is most useful when following a seriously ill patient's acid-base changes and from their directional changes infer if these changes are compensatory and likely advantageous or a new primary disorder.

Construction and Use of the Acid-Base Diagram

Figure 10-3 is constructed using logarithmic scales of pCO_2 and $[HCO_3^-]$ on the respective X and Y axes with vertical and horizontal lines at each number. Numbers for the axes are chosen so that the diagonal pH or $[H^+]$ lines intersect the junctions of the vertical and horizontal lines. One can easily construct this diagram from scratch on cross-lined graphical paper using multiples or divisors of 20, 25, 32, and 40 on the X-axis and 12, 15, 19, and 24 on the Y-axis. Diagonal pH values change by 0.10 unit at each intersection with approximate ratios of $[H^+]$ of 20, 25, 32 and 40. The oval area

Table 10-1	Approximate Combinations of Blood Bicarbonate [HCO$_3^-$] and pCO$_2$ Values with Resultant pH Values and [H$^+$] Concentrations Using the Henderson-Hasselbalch Equations. Likely Acid-Base Disorders are Identified

#	[HCO$_3^-$], mEq/L	pCO$_2$, mmHg	pCO$_2$ × 0.03	[HCO$_3^-$] /pCO$_2$ × 0.03	Log$_{10}$	Pk'	pH	[H$^+$]	Likely acid-base disorder
1	24	40	1.2	20	1.3	6.1	7.4	40	Normal
2	18	30	0.9	20	1.3	6.1	7.4	40	Chronic compensated respiratory alkalosis
3	30	50	1.5	20	1.3	6.1	7.4	40	Chronic compensated respiratory acidosis
4	30	40	1.2	25	1.4	6.1	7.5	32	Non-respiratory alkalosis
5	19	20	0.6	32	1.5	6.1	7.6	25	Acute respiratory alkalosis with partial compensation
6	7.5	20	0.6	12.6	1.1	6.1	7.20	64	Acute non-respiratory acidosis
7	28	73	2.2	12.6	1.1	6.1	7.20	64	Acute respiratory acidosis

of normality is placed at pCO$_2$ of 40 mmHg, [HCO$_3^-$] at 24 mEq/L, and pH of 7.40 and [H$^+$] of 40. The colored bands on the diagram generally cover values found in series of patients with primary disorders reported by other investigators and should not be considered rigid boundaries.[13-17]

From this site (and from any other site on the diagram), a horizontal move to the right defines an acute respiratory acidosis. A horizontal move to the left defines an acute respiratory alkalosis. A vertical upward move indicates an acute non-respiratory alkalosis; for brevity, the term non-respiratory alkalosis is often used. A

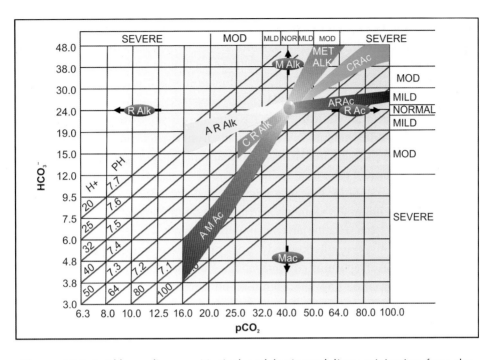

Figure 10-3 Acid-base diagram. Vertical and horizontal lines originating from the X- and Y-axes, for pCO_2 in mmHg and $[HCO_3^-]$ in mEq/L, increase and decrease in equal distances in a logarithmic scale while the intersecting diagonal lines depict arterial blood pH and $[H^+]$ intensities. Normal arterial pCO_2, pH, and $[HCO_3^-]$ are in a white oval above and to the right of the center of the diagram. Respiratory acidosis (R Ac – black oval) begins as a direct horizontal move to the right due to increasing pCO_2. Respiratory alkalosis (R Alk – black oval) begins as a direct horizontal move to the left due to decreasing pCO_2. Non-respiratory or metabolic acidosis (M Ac – black oval) begins as a direct downward move due to decreasing $[HCO_3^-]$. Non-respiratory or metabolic alkalosis (M Alk black oval) begins as a direct upward movement due to increasing $[HCO_3^-]$. Each acute disorder compensates by moving promptly towards a more neutral pH. If hypoventilation increases the pCO_2 from normal, a resultant $[HCO_3^-]$ increase, places all values in the dark blue acute respiratory acidosis (A R Ac) band. If hyperventilation decreases pCO_2 from normal, a resultant $[HCO_3^-]$ decrease places all values in the yellow acute respiratory alkalosis (A R Alk) band. With chronicity and further compensation, the values move into the chronic respiratory acidosis (green) or chronic respiratory alkalosis (orange) bands. The magenta band indicates the values found with an acute metabolic acidosis (A M Ac) while the light blue band indicates the values found with a metabolic alkalosis (M Alk). The diagram is especially useful when a patient has multiple disorders. Movement from one point to another is either compensatory or a new disorder.

vertical downward move indicates a non-respiratory acidosis; for brevity, the term metabolic acidosis is often used. If the body is able, the response to these deviations is to compensate by reducing or increasing CO_2 elimination from the respiratory system or reduce or increase $[HCO_3^-]$ excretion, primarily from the kidneys moving diagonally to attempt to return the pH to its prior value.

Without knowing the clinical setting, it is often not possible to determine the cause of the primary and compensatory movements from the location on the diagram. In one patient, a pCO_2 of 50, $[HCO_3^-]$ of 30, and pH of 7.40 could be consequent to a well compensated primary resp iratory acidosis, e.g., COPD. In another patient the same values could be due to a compensated non-respiratory alkalosis (e.g., acute vomiting and loss of stomach acid). In the pulmonary laboratory, obtaining a blood sample from a radial arterial puncture usually causes some pain, often accompanied by hyperventilation and a quick mild-to-moderate reduction in pCO_2. Thus, a patient with a chronic compensated respiratory acidosis from lung disease or severe obesity could have an arterial blood sample with a pCO_2 of 45 mmHg, a $[HCO_3^-]$ of 27 mEq/L and a pH of 7.43 due to a superimposed acute respiratory alkalosis from pain and anxiety-induced hyperventilation. When pCO_2 and $[HCO_3^-]$ are both decreased, there is less likelihood of confusing respiratory alkalosis and non-respiratory acidosis, especially when the clinical picture is taken into account. Clinically, values of pO_2 and oxyhemoglobin saturation are often helpful in making the correct diagnosis.

INTERPRETING OXYGENATION

Hemoglobin is a remarkable protein. The oxyhemoglobin association or dissociation curve[18] is also of extreme importance when considering O_2 uptake in the lung, transport of O_2-laden blood by the cardiovascular system and removal and utilization of the O_2 in the peripheral musculature and organs. The concurrent movement of CO_2 in the opposite directions is also of great importance.

It must be recognized that only a minor fraction of O_2 is removed from the inspired air at rest and during exercise. On average, exhaled air contains 4% more CO_2 and 4-5% less O_2 than room air. Therefore, at rest in normal individuals, only one-fourth of the O_2 transported by the circulatory system from the lungs to the rest of the body is utilized. The quantities of CO_2 added in the tissues are only a small fraction of the total CO_2 transported by the blood as $[HCO_3^-]$. Fortunately, these reserves can be utilized during heavy exercise or severe illnesses so that up to three-quarters of the O_2 transported in systemic arterial blood can be removed by the peripheral tissues when needed.

Figure 10-4 shows the effect of pO_2 and pH on the oxyhemoglobin saturation. In the normal lung, where PAO_2 approximates 80-110 mmHg (and PaO_2 a little less), the

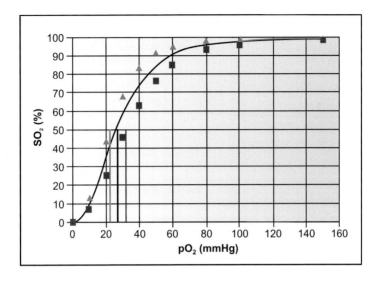

Figure 10-4 The oxyhemoglobin saturation (and desaturation) values. pO_2 values are on the X-axis and percent oxyhemoglobin saturation (SO_2) values are on the Y-axis. The three vertical lines below SO_2 of 50% indicate the P-50 values for the three pH values depicted. The black sigmoid curve shows their relationship at a pH of 7.40 ([H+] of 40) with a oxyhemoglobin saturation of 50% (P-50) designated by a short black line at pO_2 of 26.6 mmHg. The green triangles (▲) at pH 7.60 ([H+] of 25) have higher SO_2 values at those same levels of pO_2 (10, 20, 30, 40, 50, 60, 80, 100 and 150 mmHg) with a P-50 (shorter green vertical line) of 22.3 mmHg. This alkalemia is advantageous for sudden exposures to lower barometric pressure at higher altitudes or in commercial air travel where reduced pressure in the airliner cabin approximates 8,000 feet at higher cruising altitudes. (Loading of pulmonary blood is aided by the leftward shift of the curve.) It is also advantageous in any alkalemic condition as loading of hemoglobin with O_2 is facilitated. The red squares (■) at pH 7.20 ([H+] = 64) have lower SO_2 values at those same levels of pO_2 with a P-50) (longer red vertical line) of 32.3 mmHg. This acidemia is advantageous for unloading of O_2 in the peripheral musculature were acidemia secondary to the production of lactate helps O_2 unloading at the low pO_2 levels in the capillaries.

hemoglobin is 95% or more saturated with O_2. In normal subjects at rest the mixed venous pO_2 (PvO_2) approximates 40 mmHg and mixed venous oxyhemoglobin saturation approximates 70-75%. With very heavy exercise, the PaO_2 may very slightly increase or decrease, while the PvO_2 declines to 15-25 mmHg and mixed venous oxyhemoglobin saturation to 15-25%. The content of O_2 is not shown in the figure. It is dependent on the hemoglobin content of the blood. The relationship approximates

1.33–1.37 mL of O_2 per gram of fully saturated hemoglobin. With a resting hemoglobin of 15.0 g/100 mL, the content of arterial blood (CaO_2) approximates 20 g/100 mL. During heavy exercise the hemoglobin temporarily increases by about 5–7% so that the CaO_2 normally increases by that same percentage.

Reduced systemic O_2 uptake by the periphery can be due to:

A. Low arterial blood O_2 content can be due to following reasons:
    1. Low O_2 in inspired air (higher altitudes or error in inhaled gas mixtures).
    2. Inadequate ventilation (obesity; brain, sleep, or neuromuscular disorders; infiltrative lung diseases).
    3. Low ventilation/high perfusion disturbances (emphysema, chronic bronchitis, asthma, pulmonary emboli).
    4. Shunting of blood from the right heart into the left heart.
    5. Low or abnormal hemoglobin (anemia, carboxhemoglobinemia, methemoglobinemia).
B. Low cardiac output can be due to following reasons:
    1. Inadequate cardiac output (circulatory shock or heart, pulmonary vascular, and/or peripheral vascular disease).
C. Both the above mentioned conditions can be seen:
    1. High ventilation/low perfusion disturbances (emphysema, heart failure, pulmonary emboli, asthma).
D. Muscle unable to utilize delivered O_2 is seen during:
    1. Enzymatic defects (mitochondrial diseases, McArdle's syndrome).

NORMAL PAO₂ VALUES FOR MIDDLE-AGED AND ELDERLY ADULTS

The following equations of Cerveri et al.[19] are reasonable. The authors[19] obtained and promptly analyzed radial arterial blood from 194 normal seated adults from ages 40–90 years.

For ages 40–74 years, mean value for PaO_2 in mmHg = 143.6 – 0.39 × age in years – 0.56 × BMI – 0.57 × $PaCO_2$ in mmHg. SEE = 7.48.

For ages 75–90 years, mean values for PaO_2 in mmHg = 83.4 mmHg. SEE = 9.15 mmHg. The latter values were independent of BMI and $PaCO_2$. Mean ± SD values of $PaCO_2$ were 35.8 ± 3.9 mmHg.

"CORRECTIONS" FOR ALTITUDE AND TEMPERATURE

Altitude

Humans acclimatized to the lower barometric pressures of altitudes higher than sea level have large changes in their alveolar air and blood. Table 10-2 shows the approximate values of normal occupants of pressurized commercial airliners at

Table 10-2 Approximate Altitudes, Barometric Pressures (Pb), and Partial Pressures of Atmospheric (PO_2), Tracheal (PIO_2), and Alveolar O_2 (PAO_2), with Concurrent Arterial pCO_2 ($PaCO_2$) and pO_2 (PaO_2) and Saturation (SaO_2) of Long-Term Native Residents, Showing Dependency of PAO_2, PaO_2, and SaO_2 on Respiratory Exchange Ratio (R). There are no Residents at 19,000 feet or Above

Feet	Km	Pb	PO_2	PIO_2	$PaCO_2$	R = 1.0 & pH = 7.40			R = 0.8 & pH = 7.40			Site
						PAO_2	PaO_2	SaO_2	PAO_2	PaO_2	SaO_2	
0	0.0	760	160	150	40	110	99	97.5	100	90	97	Sea level
5,300	1.6	630	132	122	36	86	78	95	77	70	94	Denver
8,000	2.4	540	113	104	35	69	62	92	60	54	88	Aspen, airliners
10,000	3.0	523	110	100	34	66	59	90	57	52	86	Leadville & ski areas
13,000	4.0	440	92	83	32	51	45	81	43	38	73	La Paz, Bolivia
												Cerro de Pasco, laboratories at Pikes
14,000	4.3	425	89	79	31	48	44	80	41	37	71	Peak and Mt. Blanc
17,000	5.2	380	80	70	29	41	37	71	34	30	58	Highest habitats
19,000	5.8	350	74	64								Kilimanjaro peak
29,000	8.8	253	53	43								Mt. Everest peak

cruising altitudes, residents at altitudes up to 17,000 feet, and the challenges facing mountain climbers at even higher elevations.[20] To maintain pH values of 7.40, which are usually found in long-term high altitude residents, the $[HCO_3^-]$ values, which are not included, decline proportionally to the $PaCO_2$ values. The simplified alveolar air equation: $PAO_2 = PIO_2 - PaCO_2/R$ indicates the dependence of PAO_2 (and consequently PaO_2) on the respiratory exchange ratio (R). The R, in turn, is partially dependent on diet, while the $PaCO_2$ is dependent on the presence of acute and chronic hypo- or hyperventilation. Because hypoxia stimulates hyperventilation and a decline in $PaCO_2$, oxygenation at higher altitudes is consequently improved. However, the effects of hypoxia and fluid shifts are complex and include respiratory alkalosis and increasing hemoglobin concentration, not shown in the table. It is important to note that Andean natives have very high carbohydrate and low fat diets (increasing their R and PaO_2, while metabolism of alcohol at higher altitudes decreases the R and lowers PaO_2.

Body Temperature: Challenging Concepts

Both humans and other animals find it necessary to maintain reasonable neutrality, despite changes in core temperature. As Rahn[10] and his collaborators have pointed out, pH 7.00 is only neutral for water at 25° C. Neutrality requires that $[H^+]$ = $[OH^-]$. Or, put another way, in order to maintain neutrality, both pH and pOH must be equal. Both pH and pOH decline as temperature increases. With higher temperatures the concentration (intensity) of both the [H+] and [OH-] increase so that the [H+] is higher and the pH declines. With lower temperatures, the [H+] is lower and neutral pH rises. This same principle is also true in the animal kingdom. Rahn and colleagues[10] found that the pH of blood of cold hibernating animal when measured at cold temperatures was much higher than 7.40, but when measured at 37° C was near 7.40, the "neutral" point for animal blood, the same pH as when the animal was warm. Thus, to maintain appropriate neutrality in animals including humans, the "neutral" pH at a cold body temperatures is higher than 7.40. At very hot body temperatures the "neutral" pH is lower than 7.40. Few physicians or health professionals recall the direction and exact changes with warming or cooling. The neutral pH changes 0.0147 pH units per °C[21] while pCO_2 changes 4.4% per °C,[22] in order to maintain neutrality. Thus we physicians cannot be expected to remember the normal or neutral values of pH or pCO_2 with hypothermia or hyperthermia. Therefore it is sensible for the laboratory to report blood gases and pH values at the measured temperature of 37° C rather than to convert them or "correct" and report them at the patient's actual temperature.[22] This policy of "non-correction" avoids confusion and misunderstanding. With heating and cooling of sealed specimens of blood without bubbles it is important to note that O_2 and CO_2 contents and $[HCO_3^-]$

of blood do not change appreciably. It is only the pO_2, pCO_2, and [H+] intensities and subsequent pH measurement that change with heating or cooling.

How does this principle effect oxygenation of the blood and patient. As with CO_2 content, the O_2 content of blood not exposed to air does not change with heating or cooling. The oxyhemoglobin saturation does not change appreciably, but pO_2 of blood changes by a factor of 6% per °C.[21] The pO_2 of a sealed sample of blood (or water) rises with heating and falls with cooling. As blood gas equipment warms the blood sample properly when introduced to the machine, prior cooling or heating of the sealed blood sample does not affect the results. A hypothermic animal or patient with a normal oxyhemoglobin saturation will have a lower pO_2 (6%/°C) at a low body temperature. Therefore, for evaluating oxygenation, it is also less confusing to present all values at 37°C rather than at actual body temperature.[23]

A laboratory should always note on its reports whether or not the measured blood gas and pH values are or are not "temperature corrected."

CLINICAL EXAMPLES

Case 1

A 40-year-old male who has been vomiting for several days because of an obstructing duodenal ulcer is seen in the emergency room. The patient is not receiving O_2. An arterial blood specimen, obtained with difficulty, shows an arterial pH (pH a) of 7.44, a $PaCO_2$ of 52 mmHg, a PaO_2 of 67 mmHg and calculated $[HCO_3^-]$ of 34 mEq/L and SaO_2 of 94%. This is a primary non-respiratory or metabolic alkalosis which is partially compensated. The reduction in PaO_2 is not due to lung disease, but rather to the compensatory hypoventilation and elevated $PaCO_2$.

Case 2

An unresponsive 60-year-old woman, found in an outside doorway, is brought to the emergency room. Her rectal temperature is 30°C. The arterial blood specimen, measured at 37°C, is found to have a pH of 7.40, $PaCO_2$ of 40 mmHg and a PaO_2 of 90 mmHg. The calculated $[HCO_3^-]$ is 24 mEq/L and SaO_2 is 97%. The laboratory practice is to "correct" the blood gas values to the patient's temperature but does not so state on its report. It reports a pH of 7.50, $PaCO_2$ of 29 mmHg, a PaO_2 of 57 mmHg, a SaO_2 of 97%, and a $[HCO_3^-]$ of 24 mEq/L. The new emergency room physician is perplexed, wondering if the PaO_2 indicates hypoxemia despite the normal SaO_2 but that the pH, $PaCO_2$, and $[HCO_3^-]$ indicate a respiratory alkalosis. He calls the laboratory to find out that the measured values have been "corrected" back to the patient's body temperature. On receiving the uncorrected values the emergency room physician realizes that the patient is not hypoxemic and does not have an acid-base disturbance.

Case 3

A 35-year-old man with possible smoke inhalation is given O_2 and brought to the emergency room. Using a point-of-care instrument, an arterial blood specimen reveals a pH of 7.35, $PaCO_2$ of 45 mmHg and a PaO_2 of 225 mmHg. The calculated SaO_2 is 100% and $[HCO_3^-]$ is 24 mEq/L. This suggests that oxygenation is adequate. Fortunately a portion of the specimen was sent to the pulmonary laboratory where co-oximetry revealed a carboxyhemoglobin (COHgb) of 30% and measured oxyhemoglobin saturation of 68%. The patient is severely hypoxemic requiring treatment for carbon monoxide poisoning.

CONCLUSION

It is important to carefully obtain and identify, properly measure and report, and carefully interpret blood gases and pH. This is true whether analyses are performed at the patient's site or at a dedicated laboratory.

REFERENCES

1. Hansen JE, Simmons DH. A systematic error in the determination of blood PCO_2. *Am Rev Respir Dis.* 1977;115(6):1061-3.
2. Mahoney JJ, Harvey JA, Wong RJ, et al. Changes in oxygen measurements when whole blood is stored in iced plastic or glass syringes. *Clin Chem.* 1991;37(7):1244-8.
3. Burnett RW, Covington AK, Fogh-Andersen N, et al. Recommendations on whole blood sampling, transport, and storage for simultaneous determination of pH, blood gases, and electrolytes. International Federation of Clinical Chemistry Scientific Division. *J Int Fed Clin Chem.* 1994;6(4):115-20.
4. Severinghaus JW, Astrup P, Murray JF. Blood gas analysis and critical care medicine. *Am J Respir Crit Care Med.*1998;157(4 Pt 2):S114-22.
5. Rodkey FL, Hill TA, Pitts LL, et al. Spectrophotometric measurement of carboxyhemoglobin and methemoglobin in blood. *Clin Chem.*1979;25(8):1388-93.
6. Hansen JE, Stone ME, Ong ST, et al. Evaluation of blood gas quality control and proficiency testing materials by tonometry. *Am Rev Respir Dis.* 1982;125(4):480-3.
7. Hansen JE, Clausen JL, Mohler JG, et al. Blood gas proficiency-testing materials: a multilaboratory comparison of an aqueous solution and a fluorocarbon-containing emulsion. *Clin Chem.* 1982;28(8):1818-20.
8. Hansen JE, Casaburi R. Patterns of dissimilarities among instrument models in measuring PO_2, PCO_2, and pH in blood gas laboratories. *Chest.* 1998;113(3):780-7.
9. Sørensen SP. L Enzymstudien II. Mitteilung über die Messung und die Bedeutung der Wasserstoffionen-konzentration bein enzymatischen Prozessen. *Biochem Z.* 1909;21:131-304.

10. Rahn H, Reeves RB, Howell BJ. Hydrogen ion regulation, temperature, and evolution. *Am Rev Respir Dis*. 1975;112(2):165-72.

11. Henderson L. Blood. Yale University Press, New Haven: 1928.

12. Sun XG, Hansen JE, Stringer WW, et al. Carbon dioxide pressure-concentration relationship in arterial and mixed venous blood during exercise. *J Appl Physiol*. 2001;90(5):1798-810.

13. Albert MS, Dell RB, Winters RW. Quantitative displacement of acid-base equilibrium in metabolic acidosis. *Ann Intern Med*. 1967;66(2):312-22.

14. Arbus GS, Herbert LA, Levesque PR, et al. Characterization and clinical application of the "significance band" for acute respiratory alkalosis. *N Engl J Med*. 1969;280(3):117-23.

15. Brackett NC Jr, Wingo CF, Moren O, et al. Acid-base response to chronic hypercapnia in man. *N Engl J Med*. 1969;280(3):124-30.

16. Narins RG, Emmett M. Simple and mixed acid-base disorders: a practical approach. *Medicine (Baltimore)*. 1980;59(3):161-87.

17. Javaheri S, Kazemi H. Metabolic alkalosis and hypoventilation in humans. *Am Rev Respir Dis*. 1987;136(4):1011-6.

18. Severinghaus JW. Simple, accurate equations for human blood O_2 dissociation computations. *J Appl Physiol*. 1979;46(3):599-602.

19. Cerveri I, Zoia MC, Fanfulla F, et al. Reference values of arterial oxygen tension in the middle-aged and elderly. *Am J Respir Crit Care Med*. 1995;152(3):934-41.

20. Hultgren H. High altitude medicine. Hultgren Publications: Stanford CA: 1997; p. 550.

21. Rosenthal TB. The effect of temperature on the pH of blood and plasma in vitro. *J Biol Chem*. 1948;173:25-30.

22. Bradley AF, Severinghaus JW, Stupfel M. Effect of temperature on PCO_2 and PO_2 of blood in vitro. *J Appl Physiol*. 1956;9(2):201-4.

23. Hansen JE, Sue DY. Should blood gas measurements be corrected for the patient's temperature? *N Engl J Med*. 1980;303:41.

11 Exercise Testing

INTRODUCTION

Since patients with pulmonary and cardiovascular disorders are primarily symptomatic with exertion, exercise testing in the laboratory can assist in diagnosis, in evaluating the effect of therapeutic interventions, in adding a prescribed exercise program, and in assessing the progression or regression of disease processes over time. Exercise and levels of activity may be limited by an inactive lifestyle, obesity, endocrine, immunologic, neuromuscular, lung, or cardiovascular diseases, or by behavioral disorders. Exercise testing with gas exchange measurements can be used by the generalist, cardiologist, anesthesiologist or sports medicine specialist. However, there are times when a pulmonolgist or other physician supervises or is intimately involved in performing and interpreting such exercise testing. Therefore, a brief summary of factors relating to clinical exercise testing will be presented.[1]

PHYSIOLOGY AND PATHOPHYSIOLOGY OF EXERCISE TESTING (BRIEFLY)

Exercise, and staying alive, requires the metabolism of carbohydrate and fat with O_2 to produce CO_2, H_2O, heat and energy. To supply adequate O_2 to active muscles, the cardiac output and ventilation must increase above resting levels. When O_2 is adequately supplied from the atmosphere by the respiratory and circulatory systems to the metabolizing organs and muscles, the process is totally aerobic. When O_2 cannot be adequately supplied, anaerobic metabolism is added to the aerobic metabolism. Anaerobic processes use pyruvate and produce lactate. The resultant [H+] combines with $[HCO_3^-]$ to form H_2O and CO_2. This lactate-induced CO_2 is excess to that produced by the direct conversion of O_2 plus carbohydrate or fat to CO_2 and H_2O. In order to prevent excessive acidemia from this metabolic acidosis, the respiratory system compensates by increasing ventilation even more in order to excrete this "excess CO_2".[2] The evidence for this excess CO_2 is visible in several commonly used cardiopulmonary exercise testing (CPET) graphs.

It is also necessary to introduce the Fick principle, which is:

$$VO_2 = Q \times (CaO_2 - CvO_2),$$

Where, VO_2 is O_2 uptake in mL/min, Q = cardiac output in L/min, $CaO_2 = O_2$ content in mL/L arterial blood, and $CvO_2 = O_2$ content in mL/L in mixed venous blood.

This can also be written as:

$$VO_2 = HR \times SV \times (CaO_2 - CvO_2),$$

Where, HR = heart rate in beats/minute, SV = stroke volume in L/beat.

Since $VO_2/HR = O_2$ pulse, the O_2 pulse in mL/beat = $SV \times (CaO_2 - CvO_2)$.

O_2 pulse is obtained continuously and non-invasively during CPET from VO_2 and HR measurements. We know from invasive measurements[3,4] of CaO_2 and CvO_2 in healthy and ill individuals that SV ordinarily increases at the onset of upright exercise and remains stable throughout the remainder of exercise, except for possible mild reduction in SV at very high heart rates. We also know that, because of hemoconcentration and increase in hemoglobin concentration, CaO_2 content increases from rest to maximal exercise about 5–7%. We also know that (except in the rare patients with mitochondrial disease) mixed venous oxyhemoglobin saturation decreases from resting levels in all individuals, usually to ~15–20% in normals and ~20–25% in patients with limited cardiac output. With this knowledge we can make some assumptions and interpretations about the O_2 pulse. The O_2 pulse continues to increase in normal individuals with incremental exercise until the end or near end of maximal exercise (perhaps up to one to one and a half minutes). Therefore, with a normal arterial oxyhemoglobin saturation, a stable value for O_2 pulse strongly suggests that the patient reached their maximal extraction of O_2 (i.e., maximal reduction of SvO_2 and CvO_2) and maximal stroke volume. The only other alternative explanation is that the stroke volume was declining while O_2 extraction was increasing. If this stability in O_2 pulse lasts longer than one and a half minutes, this suggests that myocardial, pericardial, or valvular heart disease or pulmonary vascular disease is limiting stroke volume and that the exercise test has been maximal or near-maximal.

The average man can increase his resting energy requirements approximately ten-fold: More if a young athlete, less if older or inactive. If you were given the challenge of designing the human ventilatory and circulatory system to increase work load ten-fold how might you do so?

1. Would you increase ventilation and cardiac output ten-fold to increase O_2 delivery 10-fold? Air (gas) is easy to move back and forth. Blood is much denser and takes more energy to move.
2. Could you increase cardiac output 10-fold? Increase heart rate by 3 (from 60 to 180 beats per minute) and stroke volume by 3 or more times (0.1 L to 0.3 L per beat) would be 9-fold. The former is possible, the latter is not. A 30% increase in

stroke volume is reasonable; a 50% increase is possible in a few individuals; more is not realistic.

3. Could you increase the content of O_2 in arterial blood? In a liter of systemic arterial blood, 150 g of hemoglobin holds 200 mL of O_2 when it is 95–97% saturated. Increasing alveolar and arterial PO_2 adds only a trivial amount of dissolved O_2. But increasing hemoglobin concentration by 5–7% during heavy exercise is more helpful.[3]

4. Could you increase the peripheral extraction of O_2 to increase O_2 uptake? Good idea! In health, the mixed venous oxyhemoglobin saturation is ordinarily about 70% at rest, so that only 25% or so of the O_2 has been removed in passing through the healthy systemic circulation at rest. Increasing the extraction of O_2 from hemoglobin during heavy exercise so that the blood has only 20% or so oxyhemoglobin left would triple the extraction and consumption of O_2 from the same volume of blood.

5. Can one return blood from the muscles with no O_2?, that is, fully desaturated? No. The pO_2 in the capillaries must remain close to 15–20 mmHg in order for there to be adequate pressure to allow O_2 to diffuse from the capillaries to the muscle mitochondria. Therefore we cannot reduce the oxyhemoglobin saturation much lower than 15–20% (Figure 10-4). Because capillary blood is acidemic (from lactate and [H+] production), the oxyhemoglobin saturation curve shifts to the right and releases O_2 from hemoglobin more profusely. Good! So the lactate-induced acidemia is helpful in O_2 delivery to the muscle.[4]

6. Back to the lungs. With lactate-induced acidemia, the ventilatory centers are strongly stimulated to get rid of the excess CO_2. In fact, during heavy exercise, the pCO_2 of the mixed venous blood can risen to 70–80 mmHg and the mixed venous pH is very low, between 7.20–7.00.[5] With increased ventilation, the lungs increase the output of CO_2 to that the arterial blood has a much lower pCO_2 and a much higher pH than mixed venous blood.

7. The circulation must transport CO_2 from the mixed venous blood to the lungs for elimination to the atmosphere. When exercise began, the removal of O_2 from the ventilated air and movement of CO_2 from the blood to the atmosphere became a bit more efficient as the matching of lung ventilation and lung perfusion improved. Thus, ventilation from rest to maximal exercise only needs to increase about that the ten-fold we first anticipated to get rid of the metabolic CO_2 and excess CO_2. This increased removal of excess CO_2 will make the arterial pH much less acidemic than mixed venous blood (good) and usually reduces the systemic arterial pCO_2 and CO_2 content to well below resting values in order to mitigate the metabolic acidosis and keep pH near to the normal. Fortunately a good

central nervous system, ventilatory apparatus and circulatory system allow this to happen.[1,5]

8. How efficient is the system just described? In all normal individuals, within a narrow range, 10 mL/min of O_2 are required for every watt increase in external work rate ($\Delta VO_2/\Delta WR$ = 10 mL/min), whether measured during constant or incremental exercise.[6,7] When the $\Delta VO_2/\Delta WR$ is lower, this means that the amount of O_2 available from the atmosphere is inadequate, so that additional energy required to maintain the increase in work must be supplied from anaerobic metabolism (the production of lactate). While this design seems to work in healthy persons we are not sure if it works equally well in the less healthy ones.

ADVANTAGES OF THE INCREMENTAL CPET WITH GAS EXCHANGE MEASUREMENTS

If one records and reviews the cardiovascular and respiratory responses of the human suspected of having disease, during rest, mild, moderate, and heavy exercise, it is possible to learn a great deal about why the patient is symptomatic, especially if those same symptoms occur during the exercise test.[8,9] By comparing an individual's values to normal ones for a given age, gender, and body size, one can learn what system or organ limits exercise, why it does so, and how one might direct therapy.[1] One can ascertain if the patient is a safe candidate for major surgery.[10] One can prescribe exercise therapy when indicated. One can follow the effects of therapy or the disease process over time, all without radiation exposure or invasive testing. To obtain this information, one must have knowledge of the external work performed and to obtain measurements of VE and CO_2 and O_2 fractions in the expired air, plus recording of ECG complexes, heart rate and blood pressure. Estimation of oxyhemoglobin saturation is easily available using pulse oximetry. When adequate perfusion of the oximeter placed on the ear, forehead, or finger is problematic, arterial blood values may be necessary.[1]

Diagnostically, cardiopulmonary exercise testing with gas exchange measurements and especially useful in patients with suspected coronary artery disease, possible pulmonary vascular disease of any etiology or unexplained dyspnea. It may be life-saving in patients being considered for heart and/or lung transplantation, major lung resection, or in elderly patients being considered for major thoracic or abdominal surgery. It can be very useful in evaluating or guiding O_2, drug, or transplant therapy in many patients with heart or lung disease. In patients with both respiratory and cardiovascular disorders it assists in identifying the limiting disorder and the optimal therapeutic target.[1]

PERFORMING THE TEST AND DISPLAYING THE DATA

After obtaining the chief complaint and/or reason for the test, an adequate history including all current drug therapy, a brief targeted physical exam including exact height and weight, an ECG, and assuring oneself that the patient fully understands the procedures, written informed consent is obtained. Pre-exercise spirometry is highly desired; DLCO measures are often indicated. For familiarization, the patient should practice very brief mild exercise on the ergometer. The patient must be taught to communicate with the examiner using signals without verbalization. Specifically, the patient must be able to signal the occurrence of lightheadedness or chest pain or pressure. The patient must be informed and prepared if arterial or free-flowing ear capillary blood samples are to be obtained.[1]

The cycle ergometer is optimal for quantifying the work performed and for safety, since the patient can safely stop exercise at any time. When using a treadmill, the patient must learn how to exit from the moving belt when ending exercise. Quantifying external work is more difficult using the treadmill, since even minimal holding on to the examiner or handrails reduces the amount of actual external work performed. With either ergometer, continuous gas exchange measurements during periods of rest, warm-up, incremental exercise to exhaustion or safe levels, and brief recovery measurements should be made.[1,8,9]

Exercise should be incremented continuously (ramp) or every minute at a fixed increment so that the incremental portion of the study optimally lasts 8–12 minutes. For patients, cycle frequency should be maintained at 55–65 rpm; the treadmill speed should be comfortable. The increment rate (watts for the cycle and grade ± speed for the treadmill) is estimated from the information just obtained or as described elsewhere.[1]

The examiner carefully observes both the patient and the equipment-produced data as exercise progresses. It is reasonable to verbally encourage the patient. The following are reasons to stop the patient's exercise: Decreasing systolic blood pressure, increasing arrhythmias, lightheadedness, confusion, unsteadiness or symptoms compatible with myocardial ischemia. Otherwise, the operators should not have the patient stop exercise just because the heart rate exceeds 85% or 100% of that predicted by age. We routinely obtain gas exchange and ECG measures during two or more minutes of recovery. To avoid lightheadedness or increasing arrhythmias due to pooling of blood in the legs during recovery, the patient should move the pedals back and forth or in reverse at a slow rpm. After removal of the mouthpiece, the patient is promptly queried, without using leading questions, as to the reasons for stopping or symptoms at end-exercise.[1]

It is always necessary to examine the ECG tracings and all of the other data in graphical and tabular format. One must look for normal and abnormal patterns in all of the graphs and use proper predicted means and LLN values in order to reach a reasonable conclusion. Our laboratory prefers averaging peak VO_2, peak VE, peak VCO_2, peak heart rate, peak O_2 pulse, RER, and AT over a 20–30 second time period. In all cases, absolute as well as percent of mean predicted and LLN values should be considered.[11]

The VE/VCO_2 and VE/VO_2 or VCO_2/VE and VO_2/VE are usually averaged over a 60 second period. Currently, VE/CO_2 and VE/VO_2 values are most commonly displayed in CPET reports, but this may change. Lower values of VE/VCO_2 and VE/VO_2 indicate increased efficiency or decreased inefficiency of removal of CO_2 from the lung and extraction of O_2 from the inspired air. When plotted against time, their reciprocals (VO_2/VE and VCO_2/VE) obviously move in the opposite direction. It is advantageous to use VO_2/VE and VCO_2/VE, since they numerically increase when efficiency increases. Highest VO_2/VE and VCO_2/VE are higher in younger than older adults, men than women, and in very fit athletes. Thus, VO_2/VE and VCO_2/VE changes are directionally similar to those of most other CPET parameters (peak VO_2, peak O_2 pulse, anaerobic threshold and $\Delta VO_2/\Delta watts$) which indicate improvement by increasing rather than decreasing their numerical values.

INTERPRETING THE TEST

This topic is too complex to cover in detail here, but is well covered in the textbook of Wasserman et al.[1] After considering the specific value of the serial measurements of O_2 pulse, brief comments will be considered for several situations.

One of the most useful figures for evaluating cardiovascular function during rest and exercise is one displaying successive values during CPET with concurrent VO_2 values on the X-axis, HR on the primary Y-axis and VCO_2 on the secondary Y-axis. This is usually found as the center figure (number 5) in a nine-figure display. This center figure allows one to estimate the anaerobic threshold from the relationship between VO_2 and VCO_2 by the V-slope method.[1] If the scales for VCO_2 and VO_2 on the Y- and X-axes, are identical, the point of increase in slope from 45° signifies the production and release of excess CO_2, that is, the anaerobic threshold.

The figure 11-1 displays theoretical HR, VO_2, and O_2 pulse values and relationships, but not the values of an individual patient. The differently colored isopleths which radiate upward and to the right from the origin (both X and Y are zero), depict, from the VO_2 values on the X-Axis and the HR values on the Y-axis identify the theoretical (VO_2/HR) from 2 mL/beat to 24 mL/beat over a wide range. Thus on these isopleths, a single point identifies the actual VO_2 in L or mL/min, the actual HR in bpm, and the actual O_2 pulse in mL/beat. For a specific patient, an X, O, or other conspicuous symbol is placed in the upper portion of the figure at the intersection

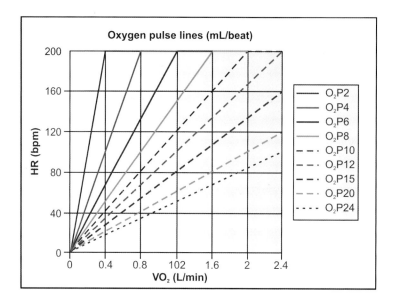

Figure 11-1 The relationships among VO$_2$ on the X-axis, HR on the Y-axis, and O$_2$ pulse (O$_2$P2) as isopleths from 2–24 mL/beat are displayed. These are not the actual values for a given patient during incremental or constant rate exercise, but demonstrate what the O$_2$ pulse values (O$_2$P2 to O$_2$P24) would be for any given VO$_2$ and HR. During a CPET, values for a normal individual move upward and to the right, across, rather than on these isopleths.

of predicted peak VO$_2$ and predicted peak HR for a normal individual of the age, gender, height and weight of the patient being tested.

The figure 11-2 displays the same VO$_2$ and HR axes as seen in the prior figure but the O$_2$ pulse isopleths are absent and replaced by the actual values during incremental exercise tests. Values are shown for five different patients, all with a predicted peak VO$_2$ of 2.0 L/min, predicted peak HR of 160 beats/min and peak O$_2$ pulse of 12.5. mL/beat (bold circle). The legend indicates the diagnosis of each patient and shows the importance of using the O$_2$ pulse values to interpret CPET studies.

Aging, Activity Levels and Nutrition

Most peak exercise values in healthy individuals are relatively stable from age 20–30 years. Thereafter, with increasing age, there is a gradual and progressive decline in peak VO$_2$, peak HR, peak O$_2$ pulse, and AT with very small decreases in highest VO$_2$/

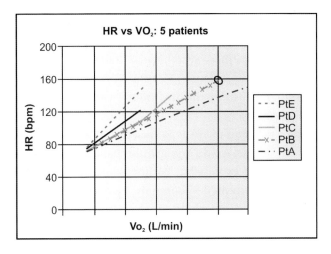

Figure 11-2 The VO_2, HR and O_2 pulse values are displayed for five different patients (A, B, C, D and E) from rest to their peak exercise. The predicted peak target value for all normal sedentary men of that same age and size is depicted as a black circle. All patients depicted start with a resting heart rate around 75 bpm. Patient A is very fit; he exceeds his predicted peak VO_2 at a lower than expected peak HR and higher than expected O_2 pulse. If the values of patient A had stopped at a considerably earlier point, i.e., well below predicted peak VO_2, the pattern would be typical for a patient on high-dose beta adrenergic blockade therapy. Such beta-blocked patients, because of their relative bradycardia, usually have higher than expected O_2 pulse values for a given work load but lower than predicted peak HR. Patient B reaches his expected peak VO_2 of 2.4 L/min, peak HR of 160 bpm and peak O_2 pulse of 15.0 mL/beat and is considered normal. Patient C starts out well and increases his O_2 pulse to approximately 10.0 mL/beat. At a HR of about 100 bpm the direction of the O_2 pulse suddenly deviates upward, continuing at approximately 10.0–10.5 mL/beat. Thus his O_2 pulse now becomes constant and no longer increases as expected. This is a typical pattern for a patient with coronary artery disease with myocardial dysfunction as myocardial ischemia develops, whether due to macro-vessel or micro-vessel coronary artery disease. Patient D values for O_2 pulse increase less than normal throughout his test. He stops exercise with an O_2 pulse of approximately 8.5 mL/beat, well below his normal predicted value for that heart rate or VO_2. From this figure alone, the cause is not clear, but might well be obstructive or restrictive lung disease with ventilatory limitation which prevents him from exercising further. If he had been able to exercise further, his peak O_2 pulse would still have been reduced as the trajectory was to the left of the peak target values. This upward deviation indicates circulatory impairment, which is nearly always due to cardiovascular disease, but could be due to severe anemia, severe carboxyhemoglobinemia or mitochondrial disease. Patient E has a persistently low O_2 pulse, with the trajectory even further to the left, reaching close to his predicted peak HR of 160 bpm, but well below his predicted peak VO_2 of 2.4 L/min, with an O_2 pulse of approximately 7 mL/beat. This pattern is typical for someone with a condition such as cardiomyopathy, valvular heart disease, pulmonary vascular disease or heart failure.

VE and VCO_2/VE (with very small increases in their reciprocals (lowest VE/VO_2 and VE/VCO_2).[1,12] These declines are slower in those who remain physically active and well-trained but are faster in those who have an inactive lifestyle. The $\Delta VO_2/\Delta WR$ remains at 10 mL/min/Watt.[1] Because FEV_1 and MVV are declining equivalently to the peak cardiovascular measures, the breathing reserve remains positive. $P(A-a)O_2$ values increase minimally.

Obesity is a major problem in Western societies. When weight gain is primarily due to increased body fat, one would expect little change in cardiovascular function. The long-held practice of expressing cardiovascular health solely in terms of mL/min/Kg is no longer warranted. Commonly, increasing weight per height is due to obesity, but in well-trained individuals much of the gain may be due to increasing muscle or lean body mass. Because carrying around excessive weight in obesity should induce a cardiovascular training effect, peak predicted VO_2 and O_2 pulse and predicted AT also increase mildly, but not in parallel with the increase in fat burden. The reference formulas of Wasserman et al. and the SHIP study are optimal in evaluating patient populations of excessive overweight or underweight.[1,13]

Cardiovascular Diseases

CPET is usually the most cost- and time-effective way to assess individuals suspected of having coronary artery disease (CAD), whether macrovascular and usually accompanied by ECG changes, or microvascular and sometimes unaccompanied by ECG changes.[14,15] Recall that ATP and VO_2 requirements continue to increase in an incremental test. The pattern commonly seen with CAD is a flattening of the $\Delta VO_2/\Delta WR$ and $\Delta VO_2/\Delta HR$ with the onset of myocardial ischemia when VO_2 supply is inadequate for normal myocardial contractility. This pattern is seen at or slightly above the AT. Since VO_2/HR (which is the same as O_2 pulse) stops increasing appropriately at this time, this means that either maximal extraction of O_2 from the periphery or, more likely, decreasing stroke volume is responsible.[1,14,15]

Systemic hypertension, unless prolonged and severe, is usually tolerated by the heart, but may result in some decline in peak VO_2 and an inordinate rise in systolic or diastolic pressures during incremental exercise. Chronotropic incompetence may be due to intrinsic heart disease or administration of high-dose beta-blockade. Ordinarily with moderate beta-blockade, the peak HR declines and O_2 pulse increases, so that the decline in the peak VO_2 is not large.[1] With long-standing systemic hypertension or cardiomyopathy of any cause, the ejection fraction may decline, indicating systolic dysfunction, or the ventricles may not relax adequately, indicating diastolic dysfunction. Both are accompanied by significant decreases in peak VO_2, peak O_2 pulse, AT, $\Delta VO_2/\Delta WR$, and mild decreases in highest VO_2/VE and VCO_2/VE.

Valvular or surgically corrected congenital heart disease may have specific patterns of abnormality reflecting right and/or left ventricular hypertrophy, shunting from right to left or left to right, and inefficient pulmonary gas exchange. Peak VO_2, peak O_2 pulse, AT, $\Delta VO_2/\Delta WR$, and VO_2/VE and VCO_2/VE are likely to be abnormal.

Heart failure due to any of the above disorders is eventually manifested by decreases in peak VO_2, peak O_2 pulse, AT, $\Delta VO_2/\Delta WR$, and VO_2/VE and VCO_2/VE.[16] More severe left ventricular failure is often manifested by oscillatory breathing, with cycles approximating 60 seconds but ranging from 40 to 120 seconds.[17,18] These cycles can be seen in plots against time of VE, VO_2, VCO_2, RER, VE/VCO_2 or VCO_2/VE, VE/VO_2 or VO_2/VE, O_2 pulse and end-tidal pCO_2 and pO_2 ($PETCO_2$, $PETO_2$), but not in HR or direct plots of VCO_2 versus VO_2. The oscillations are primarily seen at rest and usually diminish as exercise intensity increases, becoming absent above the AT. Oscillation should be visible in at least four of the above plots to be identified as oscillatory breathing.[17,18]

Combined Pulmonary and Cardiovascular Diseases

Pulmonary embolic disease and primary pulmonary hypertension due to several diseases causes both cardiovascular and pulmonary consequences. The obstruction of the pulmonary arteries by clots, the hypertrophy of the smaller pulmonary arteries, or the destruction of pulmonary capillaries all increase the workload of the right ventricle. These factors also decrease the efficiency of ventilation, since some well-ventilated volumes of the lung are not perfused. As a consequence, CO_2 and O_2 are poorly transferred between the airspaces and pulmonary circulation and ventilation is wasted.[19,20]

Patients with these disorders usually have unexplained dyspnea. Because these conditions are difficult to diagnose, ultimately fatal if untreated, and responsive to therapy, it is most important to diagnose pulmonary vascular disease early in its course. Since spirometry is often within normal limits and evidence of right ventricular hypertrophy may be limited, CPET is an important and non-invasive way to assess individuals suspected of having pulmonary vascular disease, whether embolic, idiopathic, or secondary to immunological disease. When CPET reveals low $PETCO_2$, VO_2/VE, VCO_2/VE, along with low peak VO_2 and peak O_2 pulse, pulmonary vascular disease or heart failure is likely (Note that low VO_2/VE and VCO_2/VE are equivalent to increased VE/VO_2 and increased VE/VCO_2. and increased VE vs VCO_2 slopes). These patients, despite their dyspnea, stop exercise with a large breathing reserve because of their inability to increase cardiac output satisfactorily. Hypoxemia during exercise is often not present because the primary problem is high V/Q areas rather than low V/Q areas. In perhaps 20–30% of the patients with significant pulmonary

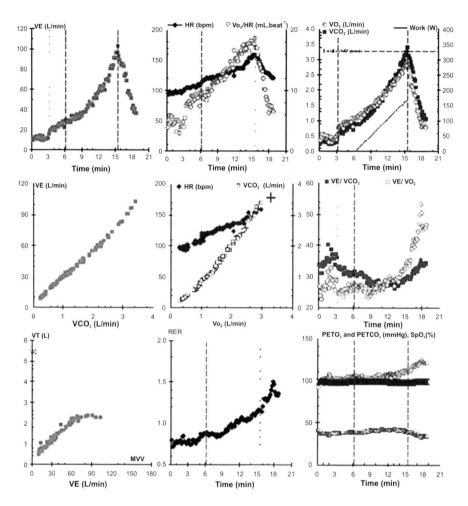

Figure 11-3A For this and the following cardiopulmonary exercise tests, the graphs of data are displayed from 1 to 9 from right to left, top to bottom. Graphs 1, 2, 3, 6, 8, and 9 all have time on the X-axis with physiological variables on the Y-axis. The vertical dotted lines in these graphs identify the start of unloaded exercise at three minutes, the change to incremental ramp exercise at six min, and the end of exercise followed by two min of recovery. On the Y-axes: Graph 1: Ventilation in L/min; Graph 2: Heart rate (HR) in beats per minutes (bpm) and O_2 pulse in (mL/beat); Graph 3: O_2 uptake (VO_2) and CO_2 output (VCO_2) in L/min and work rate in Watts; Graph 6: Ventilatory equivalents for O_2 (VE/VO_2) and CO_2 (VE/VCO_2) in BTPS/STPD; Graph 8: Respiratory exchange ratio (RER); and Graph 9: End-tidal O_2 ($PETO_2$)and CO_2 ($PETCO_2$) pressures in mmHg, oximeter hemoglobin saturation (SpO_2) in percent. Graph 4: VE versus VCO_2; Graph 5: VO_2 uptake in L/min versus HR in bpm and VCO_2 in L/min with a large **+** identifying predicted peak VO_2 and predicted peak HR; and Graph 7: tidal volume (VT) versus VE, both in L/min plus vital capacity (VC) and maximal voluntary ventilation (MVV).

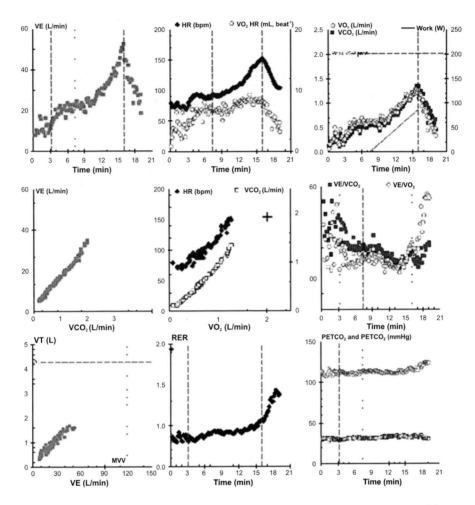

Figure 11-3B See prior figure describing graphs and symbols. This is a 65-year-old man who is 180 cm tall and weighs 72 kg. The following abnormal findings can be noted: Graph 2, peak HR is low and O_2 pulse remains flat and unchanging for the last four minutes of incremental exercise; Graph 3: peak VO_2 is low; Graph 5: AT is low; O_2 versus HR bends upward rather than continuing towards the predicted peak values, confirming the low O_2 pulse and suboptimal cardiac output; Graph 6: the lowest VE/ VCO_2 is abnormally increased; Graph 9: the $PETCO_2$ is reduced. These are typical findings in cardiovascular disease, most likely myocardial with low stroke volume and secondarily increased dead space ventilation.

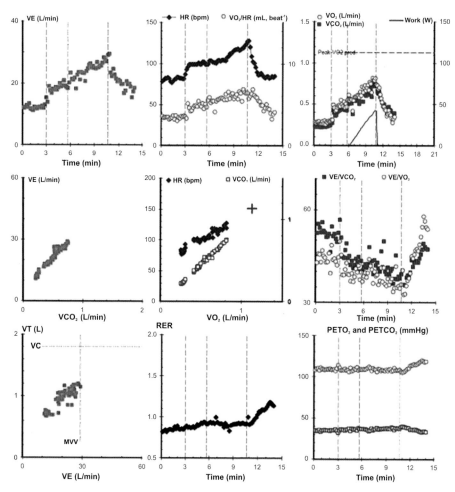

Figure 11-3C See figure 11-3A describing graphs and symbols. This is a 69-year-old woman who is 163 cm tall and weighs 60 kg. Her pulmonary function tests show obstructive lung disease with a low FEV_1, FVC, FEV_1/FVC and MVV. Look first at Graph 7, where it is clear that the patient is ventilatory limited and cannot exercise further as her peak VE reaches her MVV. In Graph 2, although the peak HR and peak O_2 pulse are low, both are increasing appropriately in Graph 5, heading towards the predicted peak values, until she can no longer exercise. Thus there is no evidence for a cardiovascular disorder. The VCO_2 does not exceed the VO_2 (Graphs 3 and 8), the AT cannot be identified (Graph 5). Since the $PETCO_2$ values are reasonably normal (Graph 9) while the lowest VE/VCO_2 and VE/VO_2 are mildly elevated (Graph 6), there is likely ventilatory inefficiency with a mild increase in dead space ventilation.

in ventilator frequency, with a large breathing reserve (difference between the MVV and peak VE). Blood pressure is not graphed, but rises with the continuing increases in HR and O_2 pulse (Graphs 2 and 5).

SIX-MINUTE WALK TEST

These tests are not diagnostic, but can be useful in evaluating therapy or following the course of an illness in patients with known pulmonary, cardiovascular, or other disorders. In the six-minute walk test, the patient is asked to cover the maximum distance in the allotted time period. Traditionally, the primary measurement made and interpreted was the distance covered walking on a level course in that time period. Now, however, oximetry, heart rate, and limited gas exchange measurements with or without telemetry are also feasible. The patient can be verbally encouraged or not, depending on the protocol requirements. In the six-minute test, running is not allowed, but the patient can stop and rest in a standing position if necessary.[30]

REFERENCES

1. Wasserman K, Hansen JE, Sue D, et al. Principles of Exercise Testing and Interpretation. (4th edn). Lippincott, Philadelphia, 2005;585.
2. Wasserman K, Van Kessel A, Burton GG. Interaction of physiological mechanisms during exercise. *J Appl Physiol*. 1967;22:71-85.
3. Stringer WW, Hansen JE, Wasserman K. Cardiac output estimated non-invasively from oxygen uptake during exercise. *J Appl Physiol*. 1997;82:908-12.
4. Stringer WW, Wasserman K, Casaburi R, et al. Lactic acidosis as a facilitator of oxyhemoglobin dissociation during exercise. *J Appl Physiol*. 1994;76:1462-7.
5. Sun XG, Hansen JE, Stringer WW, et al. Carbon dioxide pressure-concentration relationship in arterial and mixed venous blood during exercise. *J Appl Physiol*. 2001;90:1798-810.
6. Wasserman K, Whipp BJ. Exercise physiology in health and disease (State of the art). *Am Rev Respir Dis*. 1975;112:219-49.
7. Hansen JE, Sue DY, Oren A, et al. Relation of oxygen uptake to work rate in normal men and men with circulatory disorders. *Am J Card*. 1987;59:669-74.
8. Jones NL. Clinical Exercise Testing. (4th edn). Saunders, Philadelphia, 1997;259.
9. Cooper CB, Storer TW. Exercise testing and interpretation. A practical approach. Cambridge 2001;278.
10. Older P, Hall A, Hader R. Cardiopulmonary exercise testing as a screening test for perioperative management of major surgery in the elderly. *Chest*.1999;116:355-62.
11. Hansen JE, Sun XG, Yasunobu Y, et al. Reproducibility of cardiopulmonary exercise measurements in patients with pulmonary arterial hypertension. *Chest*. 2004;126:816-24.
12. Sun XG. unpublished.
13. Glaser S, Koch B, Ittermann T, et al. Influence of age, sex, body size, smoking, and beta blockade on key gas exchange exercise parameters in an adult population. *Eur J Cardiovasc Prev Rehabil*. 2010.

14. Bellardinelli R, Lacalaprice F, Carle F, et al. Exercise-induced myocardial ischemia detected by cardiopulmonary exercise testing. *Eur Heart J.* 2003;24:1304-13.

15. Chaudhry S, Arena R, Wasserman K, et al. Exercise-induced myocardial ischemia detected by cardiopulmonary exercise testing. *Am J Cardiol.* 2009;103:615-9.

16. Wasserman K, Sun XG, Hansen JE. Effect of biventricular pacing on the exercise pathophysiology of heart failure. *Chest.* 2007;132:250-61.

17. Ben-Dov I, Sietsema KE, Casaburi R, et al. Evidence that circulatory oscillations accompany ventilatory oscillations during exercise in patients with heart failure. *Am Rev Respir Dis.* 1992;145:776-81.

18. Sun XG, Hansen JE, Beshai JF, et al. Oscillatory breathing and exercise gas exchange abnormalities prognosticate early mortality and morbidity in heart failure. *J Am Coll Cardiol.* 2010;55:1814-23.

19. Oudiz RJ, Roveran G, Hansen JE, et al. Effect of sildenafil on ventilatory efficiency and exercise tolerance in pulmonary hypertension. *Eur J Heart Fail.* 2007;9:917-21.

20. Hansen JE, Ulubay G, Chow BF, et al. Mixed-expired and end-tidal CO2 distinguish between ventilation and perfusion defects during exercise in patients with lung and heart diseases. *Chest.* 2007;132:977-83.

21. Sun XG, Hansen JE, Oudiz RJ, et al. Gas exchange-induced right-to left shunt in patients with primary pulmonary hypertension. *Circulation.* 2002;105:54-60.

22. Nery LE, Wasserman K, Andrews JD, et al. Ventilatory and gas exchange kinetics during exercise in chronic airways obstruction. *J Appl Physiol.* 1982;56:1594-602.

23. Hansen JE, Wasserman K. Pathophysiology of activity limitation in patients with interstitial lung disease. *Chest.* 1996;109:1566-76.

24. Casaburi R. Long-term oxygen therapy: state of the art. *Pneumonol Allergol Pol.* 2009;77:196-9.

25. Stevenson LW, Steimie AE, Fonarow G, et al. Improvement in exercise capacity of candidates awaiting heart transplantation. *J Am Coll Cardiol.* 1995;25:163-70.

26. Older P, Hall A. Preoperative evaluation of cardiac risk. *Br J Hosp Med.* 2005;66:452-7.

27. Anderson SD. Provocative challenges to help diagnose and monitor asthma: exercise, methacholine, adenosine, and mannitol. *Curr Opin Pulm Med.* 2008;14:39-45.

28. Ben-Dov I, Sue DY, Hansen JE, et al. Bronchodilation and attenuation of exercise-induced bronchospasm by PY 108 - 068, a new calcium antagonist. *Am Rev Respir Dis.* 1986;133:116-9.

29. Casaburi R, Porszasz J. Constant work rate exercise testing: a tricky measure of exercise tolerance. *COPD.* 2009;6:317-9.

30. American Thoracic Society: Guidelines for the six-minute walk test. ATS Committee on Proficiency Standards for Clinical Pulmonary Function Laboratories. *Am J Respir Crit Care Med.* 2002;166:111–7.

12 Ethnic Differences

INTRODUCTION

Hopefully, this topic does not offend anyone. Ethnic differences are a challenging problem, filled with uncertainties. It is difficult to recommend reasonable solutions as to how to use or translate current pulmonary function reference equations derived from American, European and Australian "white" (W) populations into those for other ethnicities who comprise the great majority of us. Considering that all humans seem to have originated from common ancestors in Africa not too many millennia ago, we are nevertheless commonly divided into races and ethnicities. There is diversity not only within races and ethnicities in the United States as noted in Chapter 4 and in African populations,[1] but also between races and ethnicities.[2-4] Should we use the same reference equations for all, or can we select pulmonary function reference equations for "non-whites"?

Consider that in all studies in the United States which use the same equipment to measure populations from two or more ethnicities the FVC and TLC values are lower for individuals of the same gender, age, and height who identify themselves socially, politically, or genetically as African, African American, or "black" rather than European-American or "white." Thus, using this definition, President Barack Obama, born of a black African father and a white European-American mother, is usually considered to be "black."

A major cause of the "white-black" difference may well relate to torso/leg length.[3,4] But many other series also find that FVC and TLC values are lower in Asian than "white" populations of the same age, height, and gender. The reasons for these consistently lower volumes in Asians are not obvious. This chapter suggests a compromise for reference equations to use now, an approach which will no doubt need modifications in the future.

MEAN PREDICTED VALUES FOR ALL ETHNICITIES

In order to reliably and logically compare ethnically different populations, the separate ethnicities should be measured at the same time with the same equipment and technicians. Most reports giving reference equations for a single ethnicity do not meet this criterion. In the following paragraph are reports which meet these criteria.

In this and in most portions of this book, those of European ancestry, whether living in Europe, the America or Australia have been referred to as "white." From a large United States population measured with the same equipment and technicians, Hankinson et al. derived equations[2] for spirometric values for "Caucasians" and "Mexican-Americans" of the same gender, height and age. For given individuals, the differences between "Caucasians" and "Mexican Americans" average less than 1%. Therefore to keep our reference formulas as uncomplicated as possible, it seems reasonable to use the same predicting equations for spirometry, lung volumes and DLCO measurements for "Latins" as "whites." Thus, the same predicting equations are recommended for all individuals in North, Central, or South America, who do not identify themselves as "black" or "Asian."

Damon[3] reported FEV_1, VC, and FEV_1/VC values from nearly 400 white and 65 black Army drivers of similar standing height and ages and found black FEV_1 and FVC values were 87% of mean white values. However, the finding that sitting heights of these blacks were over 3 cm shorter than white soldiers likely accounts for a significant part of the difference. Abramovitz et al.[4] findings of white and black men and women were quite similar. Oscherwitz et al.[5] studying Asian, black, and white seamen and hospital employees, most with positive smoking histories, found FVC and FEV_1 values higher for whites than blacks and Asians but with slightly lower FEV_1/FVC values in whites. Seltzer and colleagues[6] studied thousands of men and women at several sites in the Kaiser Permanente system in California. Their use of water or wedge spirometers and technicians was randomized. When normalized for height and smoking the FVC of the blacks and Asians were both approximately 85-91% less than those of the whites. Miller et al.[7] measured scores of men and women of African and European ethnicity in Trinidad with the same equipment and technicians. Normalizing them to the same age and height, VC and TLC values were about 10% less in blacks, while DLCO values were 4% higher in black men and 11% lower in black women. Edwards et al.[8] measuring Asian Indians, Africans, and Europeans in Trinidad, converting to a common age and height, found FVC and TLC values of approximately 80% of the Europeans, DLCO values of 90-97% of the Europeans, and DLCO/VA' values of 116-121% of the Europeans. Rossiter and Weill[9] selected 97 white and 137 black workers, mostly smokers with normal chest X-rays and mild exposure to asbestos, but without dyspnea or chronic cough. In the black men, the average VC, RV, and TLC were 10% lower; the DLCO values 9% lower and the DLCO/VA' 3% higher. Thus, in these series, all measured with similar instruments regardless of ethnicity, lung volumes and DLCO were consistently lower while DLCO/VA' values were generally higher in blacks and Asians.

For the sake of simplicity, this chapter and the appendix will refer to "non-white" individuals as the "majority" of the earth's population with the symbol,

"M." Therefore for Africans, Asians and Pacific Islanders the predicting equations recommended for these "majority" or "M" populations are the same as those recommended for "blacks." Considering the wide diversity of these populations, it could be argued that this is a preposterous recommendation. But before discarding this recommendation, please consider the following:

1. Review of multiple figures in Chapters 2 and 4 shows the wide scatter of FVC and FEV_1 values within "white" series. Every series that measures lung volume values with the same equipment finds, except perhaps for those living in high mountainous or high plateau regions, higher VC and other lung volumes for the same height for individuals of European and white or Latin American adults of the same age than the "majority" or "M" ethnicities.

2. In the last half-century, there have been major changes in nutritional status in many of the majority areas of the world, so that children, rather than being 2 or 4 cm taller than their parents or grandparents, are now 4 to 8 cm taller. This change seems to be especially evident in many Asian populations. These increases may be even more marked when the youngest generation have been born in or moved from Asia to the Americas in early childhood. Although these changes likely are primarily nutritional in cause, other factors cannot be excluded. Besides these increases in height, the FVC and DLCO values for the same height seem to be higher in those who moved from Asia to the Americas in childhood or were born in the Americas.[10]

3. For the same height and age, never-smoking women have smaller FVC, FEV_1, and FEV_3 values but slightly higher FEV_1/FVC and FEV_3/FVC values than never-smoking men of the same ethnicity and area.[11] Thus, besides age, a primary determinant of FEV_1/FVC and FEV_3/FVC values in a healthy never-smoking population is likely to be their baseline FVC. This calls for a minor adjustment of FEV_1/FVC values from the W to M populations.

4. Although the RV/TLC values of women differ from men for the same age, there is no reason to believe that the RV/TLC values for the same FVC and age should differ markedly between ethnicities. Therefore, the TLC and well as FVC values will be lower in the M than the W population for the same age, height and gender.

5. Although the FVC and TLC values for the same height are higher in "whites" and "Latins" than the M populations, there is no evidence that athletic performance of the M populations are less than that of the W population. In fact, considering overall athletic performances at sporting events, the opposite may well be true. Therefore using 5% lower DLCO values for the same height, gender, and age for the M than the W population and a 5% higher DLCO/VA' values for the M than the W population are recommended.

6. For exercise testing, the recommended values should not be changed on the basis of ethnicity, since living style, nutritional status, and geography are likely much more important factors.

All reference equations can be considered compromises. Until mare complete ethinc-specific equations are developed and tested, four sets of reference equations, as given in Appendix A, are recommended: (1) for "W" women, (2) for "M" women, (3) for "W" men, and (4) for "M" men. Use the "white or W" sets for European, American, and Australian/New Zealand non-black populations. For the "majority or M" populations the sets of equations were derived as stated immediately below:

A. For FVC, FEV_6, FEV_3, ERV, IC, FRC, RV, TLC and VA'values, use 89% of the "W" values.

B. For FRC/TLC, RV/TLC, IC/ERV, %FEV_3/FEV_6, %FEV_3/FVC values, no change.

C. For FEV_1, use 90% of the "W" values, which will result in an increase in about 1% in "M" %FEV_1/FEV_6 and %FEV_1/FVC values.

D. For DLCO use 95% of the "W" values, which will result in a decrease of about 5% in "M" DLCO values and an increase of about 5.5% in "M" DLCO/VA' values.

LOWER LIMIT OF NORMAL VALUES FOR ALL ETHNICITIES

Lower and upper limit values for pulmonary function tests are also of some importance. As stated before, 95% confidence limits give some guidance but are not magical. Variability in lower limit of normal values is similar to that of mean values. For many tests, there is a tendency for variability about mean values to increase as group mean values increase due to lower ages and taller heights and for variability to decrease with individuals of shorter heights. For W individuals, these limits, derived from SEE, Syx, or RSD values, have already been given. For spirometry it is recommended that SEE, Syx, or RSD spirometric values used for W individuals also be used for M individuals. For lung volume and DLCO measurements it is recommended that the same percentage reductions or increases be used for both W and M individuals.

REFERENCES

1. Kumar R, Seibold MA, Aldrich MC, et al. Genetic ancestry in lung-function predictions. *N Engl J Med.* 2010;363:321-30.

2. Hankinson JL, Odencrantz JR, Fedan KB. Spirometric reference values from a sample of the general U.S. population. *Am J Respir Crit Care Med.* 1999;159:179-87.

3. Damon A. Negro-white differences in pulmonary function (vital capacity, timed vital capacity, and expiratory flow rate). *Human Biology.* 1966;38:380-93.

4. Abramowitz S, Leiner GC, Lewis WA, et al. Vital capacity in the negro. *Am Rev Respir Dis.* 1962;92:287-92.

5. Oscherwitz M, Edlavitch SA, Baker TR, et al. Differences in pulmonary functions in various racial groups. *Am J Epidem*. 1972;96:319-27.

6. Seltzer CC, Siegelaub AB, Friedman GD, et al. Differences in pulmonary function related to smoking habits and race. *Am Rev Respir Dis*. 1974;110:598-608.

7. Miller GJ, Cotes JE, Hall AM, et al. Lung function and exercise performance of healthy Caribbean men and women of African ethnic origin. *Q J Exp Physiol Cogn Med Sci*. 1972;57:325-42.

8. Edwards RH, Miller GJ, Hearn CE, et al. *Proc R Soc*. 1972;181:407-20.

9. Rossiter CE, Weill H. Ethnic differences in lung function: evidence for proportional differences. *Int J Epidemiol*. 1974;3:55-61.

10. Korotzer B, Ong S, Hansen JE. Ethnic differences in pulmonary function in healthy nonsmoking Asian-Americans and European-Americans. *Am J Respir Crit Care Med*. 2000;161:1101-8.

11. Hansen JE, Sun XG, Wasserman K. Ethnic- and sex-free formulae for detection of airway obstruction. *Am J Respir Crit Care Med*. 2006;174(5):493-8.

13 Final Interpretation

GENERAL REMARKS

Viewing patients' patterns on tracings help us in reviewing the patients' performance and quality of the pulmonary function test. Comparing measured values to the mean and variability of reference values are also important. In this chapter we will look primarily at numbers, but we must remember to also look at the tracings. Please refer to Appendix A for the reference equations and values selected. Many other reference equations are available in Appendix B if you wish to refer to them.

Pulmonary function tests may not be the final answer, but they may offer considerable assistance in diagnosis, assessing severity, and assessing therapy. In screening examinations, the subject may have little or no symptoms or findings, and may or may not have been exposed to noxious particulates, fumes or chemicals. Analysis of the pulmonary function tests may, on occasion, yield very specific diagnoses, e.g., upper airway obstruction, or severe obstructive lung disease, but most commonly, it adds to the information already available to the clinician who requested the pulmonary function tests. Sometimes it adds alternate and unexpected diagnoses; sometimes it refutes diagnoses. When a patient has two or more disorders, figures and tables such as those presented may be of limited value, or very helpful. Reviewing the patient's history and physical examination or obtaining serial pulmonary function tests is worthwhile. If the patient has pain, weakness, or difficulty in performing the initial tests, they may need to be repeated a short time later. Serial tests over months or years may be important in understanding the progression or regression of a disease process or the responses to therapy.

ATS/ERS TASK FORCE RECOMMENDATIONS

In 2005, the American Thoracic Society and European Respiratory Society published a joint position paper on interpretative strategies for lung function testing[1] which was a revision of the American Thoracic Society recommendations of 1991.[2] Their algorithm[1] defined a method for narrowing etiologies of diagnostic possibilities. The committee added the comment, "the flow chart was not suitable for assessing the severity of upper airway obstruction." Their algorithm with minor modifications is shown in figure 13-1.

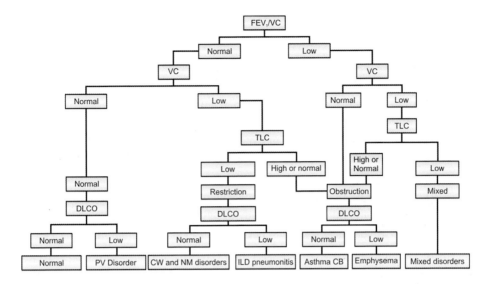

Figure 13-1 Modified 2005 ATS/ERS task force algorithm for interpreting lung function testing. Abbreviations: CB = chronic bronchitis; CW = chest wall; DLCO = diffusing capacity for carbon monoxide; FEV_1 = forced expiratory volume in one second; ILD = interstitial lung disease; NM = neuromuscular; PV = pulmonary vascular; TLC = total lung capacity; VA′ = effective alveolar volume; VC = vital capacity.

NEW RECOMMENDATIONS, INCLUDING EVALUATING OBESITY EFFECTS ON LUNG FUNCTION

In addition to the ATS/ERS approach, it is reasonable to consider additional or alternative ways of interpreting pulmonary function tests clinically. No figure or table can be expected to act as a complete "cook book." Nevertheless these aids may reduce the likelihood of going too far astray. This is true particularly when the patient has more than one disorder.

In our pulmonary function laboratory experience, the most common patient disorder other than intrinsic lung disease is obesity. It affects over one-third of all the patients coming to our laboratory. This high prevalence is likely experienced in many other centers. There are at least two simple mathematical ways to estimate the severity of obesity in adults. Both methods have the disadvantage that well-muscled individuals may have increased values due to increased lean body mass rather than fat. Overall obesity is commonly assessed by calculating the body mass index (BMI). The BMI is calculated by dividing the weight in kg by height in meters squared. BMI values for underweight, normal, overweight, obese, and morbidly or very obese are: < 20, 20–25, 25–30, 30–40, and >40 kg/m^2, respectively.

A second way to estimate the severity of obesity is to relate height in centimeters less 100 to weight in kg Normal rather than average diet and exercise in many Western societies results in an adult height in cm which exceeds the weight in kg by 100. Thus, the difference between height in cm and weight in kg plus 100 indicates the deficit or excess body weight in kg. Thus, regardless of height,

- If 20 kg underweight: height in cm = body weight in kg + 120, then the BMI ~ 17
- If 10 kg underweight: height in cm = body weight in kg + 110, then the BMI ~ 20
- If normal weight: height in cm = body weight in kg + 100, then the BMI ~ 24
- If 15 kg overweight: height in cm = body weight in kg +85, then the BMI ~ 30
- If 30 kg overweight: height in cm = body weight in kg by 70, then the BMI ~ 35
- If 55 kg overweight: height in cm = body weight in kg by 45, then the BMI ~ 40
- If 40 kg overweight: height in cm = body weight in kg by 60, then the BMI ~ 45

Lung volumes are often more affected by thoracic and abdominal obesity than by lower abdominal and extremity obesity. With obesity, the ERV usually decreases much more than the VC, IC, RV or TLC. The IC/ERV ratio approximates 1.5 in adults with BMI < 20; 2.0 to 3.0 in adults with BMI of 20 to 30; and 3.0 to 4.0 in adults with BMI of 30 to 35. With BMI values of 35 or more, the IC/ERV may increase to 10/1 or more with ERV values of 100 mL or less. Because obesity increases in most populations with aging, the IC/ERV also gradually increases with aging. Thus, in patients with complaints of shortness of breath who are referred for pulmonary function testing, the effects of obesity must be assessed by measuring the lung volumes.

Table 13-1 is proposed as a way of comparing key pulmonary function data and clinical conditions. The reader may be upset because there are a range of findings for a specific disorder, but that is reality. For example, a diversity of findings may be present in asymptomatic smokers or patients with interstitial lung disease.

- Row # 1 gives a grade for obesity which should be added to the grades for each condition given in later rows in the table.
- For row # 3, an asymptomatic smoker, the FEV_1/VC and FEV_3/VC are most likely to be above the lower limit of normal or mildly abnormal; the VC may be normal, decreased, or increased; the RV/TLC may be increased or normal; and the DLCO and DLCO/VA' may be decreased or normal.
- For row # 9, interstitial lung disease, many have a FEV_1/VC which is considerably higher than predicted mean; others do not. Some retain a normal RV/TLC, while in others the RV/TLC is elevated. Some have a low VC, a low DLCO, and a low DLCO/VA. Others have equal reductions in VC and DLCO, with a normal DLCO/VA'. Others may have with a low normal or mildly reduced VC, but a large reduction in DLCO and a low DLCO/VA'.

Table 13-1 Usual Pulmonary Function Test Findings Accompanying the Following Disorders. Rows (#) 2 to 20 are Without Obesity; i.e., BMI < 30, or Height in cm > Weight in kg + 85, or IC/ERV < 4

#	Diagnosis	$FEV_1/VC \pm FEV_3/VC$	VC	BD response	RV/TLC	VA'/TLC	DLCO	DLCO/VA'
1	Obesity (with BMI > 30 to 50 or IC/ERV > 4 to 10) add the following to each of the rows below	0	↓↓↓ to ↓	0	0	↓	0 to ↑↑	↑ to ↑↑
2	Normal	0	0	0	0	0	0	0
3	Asymptomatic smoker	↓ to 0	↓ to ↑	0 to ↑	0 to ↑	↓ to 0	↓ to 0	↓ to 0
4	Asthma, acute episode	↓↓↓	↓↓↓	↑ to ↑↑	0 to ↑↑	↓ to ↓↓↓	↓↓ to ↑↑	↓ to ↑
5	Asthma, chronic, moderate	↓↓ to 0	↓ to ↑	↑ to ↑↑↑	0 to ↑↑	↓↓ to ↓↓↓	↓ to ↑	0 to ↑
6	Chronic bronchitis	↓ to 0	↓ to ↑	0 to ↑↑	↓ to ↑	↓ to ↑↑	↓ to ↑	↓ to ↑
7	Emphysema	↓↓↓ to ↓	↑ to ↑↑↑	0 to ↑↑	↑ to ↑↑↑	↓↓↓ to ↓↓	↓↓↓ to ↓	↓↓↓ to ↓
8	Bronchiectasis	↓↓ to 0	↓ to 0	0 to ↑↑	↓ to ↑	↓ to 0	↓ to ↑	↓ to ↑
9	Interstitial lung disease	0 to ↑↑	↓↓↓ to 0	0 to ↑	0 to ↑	↓↓ to 0	↓↓↓ to↓	↓↓↓ to 0
10	Connective tissue disease	0 to ↑	↓↓↓ to 0	0 to ↑	0 to ↑	↓↓ to 0	↓↓↓ to ↓	↓↓↓ to 0
11	Asbestosis	↓ to 0	↓↓↓ to ↓	↓ to 0	↓ to ↑	↓↓ to 0	↓↓↓ to ↓	↓↓↓ to ↓

Contd...

Contd...

12	Other pneumoconiosis	→ to 0	↓↓ to ↓	0	→ to ↑	↓↓ to 0	↓↓ to →	↓↓ to 0
13	Immunological lung disease	→ to ↑	→ to 0	0	→ to ↑	↓↓ to 0	↓↓↓ to →	↓↓↓ to 0
14	Sarcoidosis	→ to ↑	↓↓ to 0	0 to ↑	0 to ↑	→ to 0	↓↓ to →	↓↓ to →
15	Pneumonia or infiltrates	→ to 0	↓↓↓ to →	0 to ↑	0 to ↑	→ to 0	↓↓ to →	↓↓ to 0
16	Pulmonary infarction/ bleeding	→ to 0	→ to 0	0	0 to ↑	→ to 0	↓↓ to ↑	→ to ↑
17	Pulmonary vascular diseases infarction	0	→ to 0	0	0	0	↓↓↓ to 0	↓↓↓ to 0
18	Heart failure	↓↓ to 0	↓↓↓ to →	0 to ↑↑	0	↓↓ to 0	↓↓ to 0	→ to ↑
19	Lung malignancies	0	↓↓↓ to 0	0	0	→ to 0	↓↓ to →	→ to 0
20	Chest wall, pain, effusions, weakness	→ to 0	↓↓↓ to →	0	→ to ↑	→ to 0	↓↓↓ to →	0

Abbreviations: BD = aerosolized bronchodilator drug; BMI = body mass index; ERV = expiratory reserve volume; FEV_1 and FEV_3 = forced expiratory volume in one and three seconds; RV = residual volume; TLC = total lung capacity; DLCO = transfer factor for carbon monoxide; VA' = effective alveolar volume; VC = vital capacity; 0 = within normal limits; ↓, ↓↓, and ↓↓↓ indicate, respectively, mild, moderate, and severe decrease; ↑, ↑↑, and ↑↑↑ indicate, respectively, mild, moderate, and severe increase.

ASSIGNING SEVERITY

Assigning severity to pulmonary function tests remains arbitrary, without universal consensus. Severity can be assigned to individual tests, e.g., FEV_1 or DLCO or other test, but severity is probably best assigned to the combination of tests. The US Social Security administration considers FEV_1 values and DLCO values below 40% of mean predicted as severe and compensable.[3] The use of 80% of predicted as a dividing line between normal and abnormal is outmoded. Generally, the author prefers grading along a continuum like the following:

FEV_1/FVC and FEV_3/FVC

- For smoker, consider reporting spirometric lung age as described in Chapter 4.
- Use for identifying obstruction, but not in isolation for grading severity.
- If FEV_3/FVC is a greater percentage away from predicted mean than FEV_1/FVC, airway obstruction is likely predominantly of smaller airways.
- Do not use $FEF_{25-75\%}$

FEV_1 or Ventilatory Ability: Possible Approximate Modifiers

- Normal, well above average: >1.65 RSD above predicted mean: Grade A.
- Normal, better than average: > 1.00 RSD above predicted mean: Grade B.
- Normal, average: 0.5 RSD-1.0 RSD above and below predicted mean: Grade C.
- Within normal limits: 1-1.5 RSD below predicted mean: Grade D.
- Probably decreased: 1.5-1.65 RSD below predicted mean: Grade E.
- Mildly decreased: <1.65 RSD below predicted mean to > 65% below predicted mean.
- Moderately decreased: 45-65% of predicted mean.
- Severely decreased: below 45% of predicted mean.
- Modifying adjectives can be combined, e.g., mildly to moderately decreased for about 65% below predicted mean.

TLC

- Increased: greater than 1.65 RSD above or 120% of predicted mean.
- Normal: Between 1.65 RSD above and 1.65 RSD below predicted mean. Alternatively, between 80% and 120% of predicted mean values.
- Mildly decreased: below 1.65 RSD or between 70% and 80% of predicted mean.
- Moderately decreased: 50-70% of predicted mean.
- Severely decreased: below 50% of predicted mean.

DLCO (TLCO) and DLCO/VA' (TLCO/VA' or KCO) for All Adults

- Increased: above 1.65 RSD or 125% of predicted mean.
- Normal: between 75% and 125% of predicted mean.

- Possibly increased: from 1.0-1.65 RSD or 115-125% of predicted mean.
- Mildly decreased: below 1.65 RSD and between 65-75% of predicted mean.
- Moderately decreased: 45-65% of predicted mean.
- Severely decreased: below 45% of predicted mean.

Combined Obstructive and Restrictive Defects

When FEV_1 is decreased from more than one cause, one can use ventilatory severity as discussed in paragraph (**FEV$_1$ or ventilatory ability: Possible Approximate Modifiers**) The discrimination whether the defect is primarily obstructive or restrictive is sometimes difficult and even arbitrary. Ordinarily, mild plus mild = moderate; moderate plus mild = severe. When both obstructive and restrictive defect are present, list what you believe to be dominant first, or divide the defect into components, e.g., severe ventilatory defect due to moderate obstructive defect and mild restrictive defect.

Combinations with Vascular Defects

When either obstructive or restrictive defects are combined with vascular defects, the severity of the combined disorders usually exceeds that of each component. For example, a moderate ventilatory defect and a moderate vascular defect should usually be considered an overall severe disorder; while a severe restrictive defect and severe vascular defect should be considered an overall very severe disorder.

USEFUL PHRASES TO CONSIDER IN YOUR INTERPRETATIONS

1. Selection of ethnicity was by the patient.
2. Weight could not be measured and was therefore estimated.
3. Shoeless height could not be obtained.
4. Because of spinal deformity and/or the inability to obtain a standing height, the arm span was substituted for standing height in predicting equations.
5. The patient had significant discomfort during the testing so that recorded values may not reflect the patient's best possible values.
6. There was difficulty in communicating with the patient so that the recorded values may not reflect the patients best possible values.
7. The age or size of the patient is beyond the range of the populations used to establish the reference values. As such, predicted values are less reliable.
8. Despite the low vital capacity, the normal inspiratory capacity with a low expiratory volume is typical of obesity rather than intrinsic lung disease.
9. The low expiratory reserve volume is typical of obesity.
10. The negligible expiratory reserve volume is typical of very severe obesity.

11. The contour of the flow volume loops suggests.
12. The reduced inspiratory flow may be due to reduced patient effort or the reduced inspiratory flow is not due to reduced patient effort.
13. The actual MVV is below that of the actual $FEV_1 \times 40$ which may be due to.
14. The actual MVV is well above the actual $FEV_1 \times 40$, which is often seen in patients with interstitial lung disease or increased elastic recoil.
15. The patient received aerosolized bronchodilator shortly before coming to the laboratory making the determination of bronchodilator effect uncertain.
16. After aerosolized albuterol (or other) administration, there is a minimal (< 6%) or mild (6-12%) or moderate (12-24%) or marked (> 24%) improvement in FEV_1 (and FEV_3 and/or FEV_6 and/or FVC). These changes are consistent and statistically significant.
17. After aerosolized albuterol (or other) administration there is no significant improvement in FEV_1 or FEV_3. The lack of bronchodilator response does not preclude its use if clinically indicated.
18. The patient was unable to attain an adequate inspiratory vital capacity during the single breath test. Therefore the VA' and TLC may be underestimated.
19. The inspiratory vital capacity maneuver in the single breath test was appropriate. The low VA'/TLC indicates maldistribution of ventilation.
20. The DLCO and DLCO/VA' values are based on an assumed, not measured, hemoglobin concentration.
21. Some of the requested measurements could not be obtain due to.

If indicated, please reschedule the patient for additional testing at a later date or we have rescheduled the patient for further testing on.

PULMONARY LABORATORY REPORT FORMAT

Top of the Report

Laboratory name, address and contact information:
Referring MD and contact information:
Reason for referral or suspected diagnosis:
Name, gender, date of birth, identity number, contact information
Measured shoeless height and uncluttered weight (cm and kg preferred)

Next: Predicted and Patient Values

Full Report Section 1: Spirometry and Lung Volumes (all best or average values):
Columns titled: (a) Measure, unit; (b) predicted mean; (c) ULN/LLN (LLN preferred); (d) pre-bronchodilator value; and (e) post-bronchodilator value

Rows titled: SVC, L; FVC, L; FEV_1, L; FEV_3, L, FEV_6, L, $\%FEV_1/FEV_6$ or $\%FEV_1/FVC$; $\%FEV_3/FEV_6$ or $\%FEV_3/FVC$; MVV, L/min; IC, L; ERV, L; FRC, L; RV, L; TLC, L; and RV/TLC. Add single best flow-volume tracing if possible.

Full Report Section 2: Single Breath DLCO; Single Breath O_2 Tests; Oximetry; and/or Arterial Blood Findings or Other

Columns titled: (a) Measure, unit; (b) predicted mean; (c) ULN/LLN; and (d) pre-bronchodilator value.

Rows titled: Hemoglobin (measured or estimated); IVC, L; VA', L; DLCO, mL/min/mmHg; DLCO/VA'; VA'/actual TLC; SBO_2, $\%\Delta N_2/L$; or other.

Partial report: May include only portions of the above or other specific tests.

Next: Sources and Abbreviations

Identify abbreviations. Give first author and year of all predicting equations. State whether predicted or measured DLCO values are modified by abnormal hemoglobin concentration.

Next: Physician Interpretation and Comments

Include relevant technician's observations regarding test quality, pain, inability to measure height or weight etc. He can add spirometric grades and/or lung age, if the person is a smoker. Add table with key results of prior tests. Interpreting physician signature, name and identity number also needs to be done.

Bottom of Page

Patient identification, date of test.

CONCLUSION

The following statement is meant to be humorous: When all else fails, look at the tracings!! Seriously, tracings should be reviewed by the interpreter. If the numbers and the tracings do not seem to fit, then re-examine both carefully. The best laboratories, best equipment, and best technicians can still make errors. It is our responsibility to detect and correct errors before a report is sent to the patient's health care provider.

REFERENCES

1. Pelligrini R, Viegi G, Brusasco V, et al. Interpretative strategies for lung function tests. *Eur Respir J.* 2005;26(5):948-68.
2. Lung Function Testing: Selection of Reference Values and Interpretative Strategies. American Thoracic Society. *Am Rev Respir Dis.* 1991;144(5):1202-18.
3. Disability Evaluation Under Social Security (Blue Book- September 2008) 3.00 Res-piratory System: Adult; online at http://www.socialsecurity.gov/disability/professionals/blue-book/3.00-Respiratory-Adult.html. Last accessed Mar 8, 2010.

CHAPTER 14 Ten Cases to Consider and Analyze with Questions and Answers

Case 14-1

This is a case of 58-year-old black man, who has recently become short of breath without apparent reason. He has smoked half packs of cigarettes per day and is still smoking. No known occupational exposure. Figure 14-1 shows his flow-volume tracing and table 14-1 gives his pulmonary laboratory data.

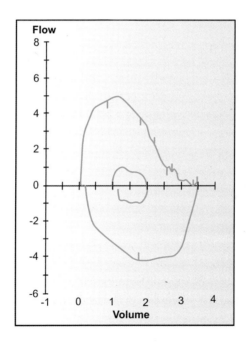

Figure 14-1 Flow-volume tracing: Volume in liters on the X-axis; Expiratory flow in liters/sec is positive while inspiratory flow is negative. Tidal volume breathing is in the center. Tracing is reasonably normal for a 58-year-old male.

Table 14-1	Selected Pulmonary Function Values for Patient 1			
Name	#	Yrs	cm	kg
Patient 1	1	58	175	85.5
Measure, units	Mean		LLN/ULN	Actual
SVC, L	4.13		3.16	3.47
FVC, L	4.13		3.16	3.50
IC, L	3.10			2.07
ERV, L	1.03			1.43
FRC, L	3.00			3.56
RV, L	1.97		**2.76**	2.13
TLC, L (LLN)	6.10		4.88	5.63
TLC, L **(ULN)**	6.10		**7.32**	5.63
RV/TLC	0.32		**0.41**	0.38
FEV_1, L	3.22		2.41	2.80
FEV_3, L	3.77		2.87	3.36
%FEV_1/FVC	78.1		68.6	80.0%
%FEV_3/FVC	91.2		86.2	96.0%
MVV, L/min	129		96	81
SBO_2 ^%N_2/L **(ULN)**			**2.3**	2.7
IVC, L				3.20
VA', L	6.10			5.40
VA'/TLC	0.95		>0.85	0.96
DLCO, mL/min/torr	29.3		22.0	8.1
DLCO/VA'	-4.81		3.61	1.50

ULN: Upper limit of normal; LLN: Lower limit of normal.

Question 14-1-1: Considering the patient's normal spirometry and lung volumes, is there any further measurement, which is necessary?

Answer: Yes, the single breath DLCO is another important measurement which has to be considered.

Question 14-1-2: Why are the patient's DLCO and DLVCO/VA' so low?

Answer: This is an important question which is not answered by these pulmonary function tests alone. The patient clearly shows the loss of pulmonary capillary bed without having significant obstructive or restrictive lung disease. Pulmonary vascular disease, a distinct possibility, could be idiopathic, or due to pulmonary emboli or secondary to pharmaceuticals or immunological disorders.

Question 14-1-3: What further investigations might be helpful?

Answer: Start with complete history and physical examination, radiographs of the chest, ECG, Cardiopulmonary exercise tests, and echocardiogram.

Case 14-2

This is a case of 60-year-old black woman, who complained of shortness of breath. She suffered from increasing obesity and increasing abdominal girth without jaundice. She had occasional wheezing. She had smoked about five pack-years of cigarettes. She denied chest pain. Additional information is that her end-tidal CO_2 measured during the single breath O_2 maneuver was 8% or about 56 mmHg. While breathing room air, her ear oximeter reading is 93%. Table 14-2 shows her pulmonary laboratory data; figure 14-2A shows her flow-volume tracing; figure 14-2B shows her single breath oxygen test.

Table 14-2	Selected Pulmonary Function Values for Patient 2			
Name	#	Yrs	cm	Kg
Patient 2	2	60	163	150.5
Measure, units	Mean		LLN/**ULN**	Actual
SVC, L	2.87		2.17	1.19
FVC, L	2.87		2.17	1.16
IC, L	2.15			1.10
ERV, L	0.72			0.09
FRC, L	2.42			1.07
RV, L	1.70		**2.31**	0.96
TLC, L (LLN)	4.57		3.66	2.17
TLC, L (**ULN**)	4.57		**5.48**	2.17
RV/TLC	0.37		**0.46**	0.45
FEV_1, L	2.25		1.68	0.91
FEV_3, L	2.62		1.98	1.09
%FEV_1/FVC	78.4		68.9	78%
%FEV_3/FVC	91.3		86.8	94%
SBO_2 ^%N_2/L (**ULN**)			**6.9**	1.9
IVC, L				1.10
VA', L	4.57			2.3
VA'/TLC	0.95		>0.85	1.06
DLCO, mL/min/torr	20.4		15.3	13.9
DLCO/VA'	4.46		3.35	6.04

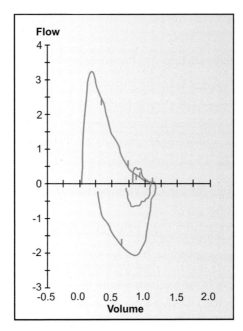

Figure 14-2A Flow-volume tracing. Note that scale differs markedly from Figure 14-1. Tidal breathing is in the center. Note the minute volume between resting exhalation and forced exhalation, which is the expiratory reserve volume (ERV).

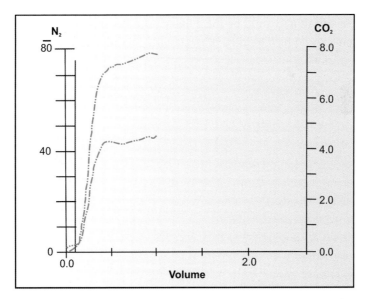

Figure 14-2B Single breath oxygen test tracings. Full inhalation of O_2 followed by slow exhalation. The percent nitrogen of exhalate (lower tracing) is on the left Y-axis; the percent CO_2 of exhalate (higher tracing) is on the right Y-axis.

Question 14-2-1: Which lung volumes or capacities are proportionally reduced the most?

Answer: The ERV reduction is classical for extreme obesity. The patient's BMI is 57 kg/m^2.

Question 14-2-2: Are the IC and VC decreased more than expected due to morbid obesity alone?

Answer: Yes, unless the obesity is extreme, the IC is usually close to or above the mean predicted in obesity. Thus, this considerable reduction in IC indicates an additional process.

Question 14-2-3: The IVC for the DLCO maneuver is 1.1 L, equivalent to the FVC values. Why is the VA' only 2.3 L?

Answer: Because the measured TLC, calculated by adding the IC of 1.10 L from spirometry and the FRC of 1.07 L by N_2 washout are 2.2 L. The author cannot expect the VA' volume to exceed the TLC measurement by any significant amount unless there is an error in one or more measurements.

Question 14-2-4: Why is the DLCO/VA' increased?

Answer: This ratio is increased because the VA' (and TLC) are well-perfused and the pulmonary capillaries are probably well-filled with blood, even at rest.

Question 14-2-5: Beside morbid obesity, what diagnoses and treatment would you consider?

Answer: High end-tidal CO_2 and low SpO_2 indicate CO_2 retention and hypoxemia. Congestive heart failure would be most likely. After treatment with O_2 therapy and diuretics there should be a marked diuresis with decrease in weight and increase in IC and FVC.

Case 14-3

This 59-year-old white male has 40 pack-years of cigarette smoking and is still smoking. He denies cough, sputum, wheezing, and dyspnea. Review tables 14-3A and B, and figure 14-3.

Table 14-3A	Selected Pulmonary Function Values for Patient 3			
Name	#	yrs	cm	kg
Patient 3	3	59	180	66.4

Measure, units	Mean	LLN/**ULN**	Pre-BD	Post-BD
SVC, L	4.89	3.92	5.22	5.67
FVC, L	4.89	3.92	5.20	5.52
IC, L	3.67		2.69	3.14
ERV, L	1.22		2.53	2.53
FRC, L	3.59		5.59	
RV, L	2.37	**3.16**	3.06	
TLC, L (LLN)	7.26	5.81	8.28	
TLC, L (**ULN**)	7.26	**8.71**	8.81	
RV/TLC	0.33	**0.42**	0.37	
FEV$_1$, L	3.72	2.91	3.59	3.81
FEV$_3$, L	4.43	3.53	4.50	4.66
%FEV$_1$/FVC	76.1	66.6	69.0	
%FEV$_3$/FVC	90.7	85.6	86.5	
MVV, L/min	149	116	105	121
SBO$_2$ ^%N$_2$/L (**ULN**)		**1.5**	2.6	
IVC, L			4.80	
VA', L	7.26		7.80	
VA'/TLC	0.95	>0.85	0.94	
DLCO, mL/min/torr	31.7	23.8	20.4	
DLCO/VA'	4.37	3.28	2.60	

Table 14-3B Values for 3 Trials Pre- and Post-BD		
FEV$_1$	Pre-BD	Post-BD
Trial 1	3.51	3.78
Trial 2	3.59	3.79
Trial 3	3.53	3.81
t-test p =		0.0003
Rank order p =		0.05
FEV$_3$		
Trial 1	4.37	4.64
Trial 2	4.50	4.66
Trial 3	4.43	4.61
t-test p =		0.004
Rank order p =		0.05
FVC		
Trial 1	5.2	5.36
Trial 2	5.19	5.52
Trial 3	5.2	5.46
t-test p =		0.003
Rank order p =		0.05

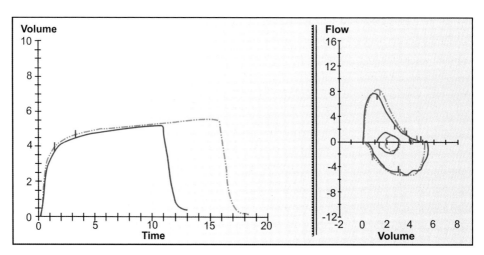

Figure 14-3 The volume-time tracings are on the left; the flow-volume tracings are on the right. The best pre-BD tracings are darker solid lines; the best post-BD tracings are lighter dotted lines.

Question 14-3-1: Why does the patient has such a large ERV?

Answer: The large ERV is typical for thin patients with large lung volumes.

Question 14-3-2: Does the patient shows the evidence for obstructive lung disease?

Answer: The %FEV_1/FVC and %FEV_3/FVC are both decreased but slightly above the 95% LLN confidence limits. The TLC and RV/TLC are increased. The DLCO and DLCO/VA' are both well below the 95% confidence limits. The below normal flows, even though not below the 95% confidence limits, the increased lung size, and loss of pulmonary capillaries (low DLCO and DLCO/VA') are strong evidence for pulmonary emphysema.

Question 14-3-3: Note that the patient's pre-BD FEV_1 actual/predicted is 3.59/3.72 or 97% of predicted FEV_1. Does that exclude airway obstruction?

Answer: The answer is certainly not. There is high variability in FEV_1 and FVC values in a population of the same ethnicity, gender, age and height. Despite the guidelines of some authorities, it is unreasonable to exclude airway obstruction just because the FEV_1 value is near mean predicted.

Question 14-3-4: Check the best pre-BD and best post-BD values in table 14-3A. Using the ATS/ERS guideline criteria, does the patient meet the criteria for bronchodilation by the administered aerosol?

Answer: The answer is No. The patient does not meet the ATS/ERS guideline criteria for bronchodilation. Although the increase in FEV_1 and FEV_3 are 220 mL, 160 mL, and 320 mL, respectively, the percentage increases are 6%, 4%, and 6%, respectively, not 12% as required by the guidelines. Because the ATS/ERS guidelines require both a 200 mL and 12% increase in FEV_1, this study does not meet their guideline for "clinical responsiveness".

Question 14-3-5: Check again the three spirometric trials pre- and post-BD in table 14-3B noting especially the t-test and rank order test p values. Are there consistent and statistically significant increases in FEV_1, FEV_3 and FVC post-BD?

Answer: Yes, there is a consistent and statistically significant increase in the FEV_1, FEV_3 and FVC post-BD values.

Question 14-3-6: Do you think that the physician who interprets pulmonary function tests, but does not care for the patient, should report whether or not a bronchodilator response is "clinically significant" based on population-based ATS/ERS guidelines?

Answer: In the author's opinion, the interpreter should note the percentage increases and state whether or not the responses are consistent and/or statistically significant. The determination of whether or not a response is clinically significant should be determined by the clinician caring for the patient.

Case 14-4

This 64-year-old non-obese black man has a 45 pack-year history of cigarette smoking, but stopped six months ago. He has a productive cough, wheezes, and is short of breath. He had no bronchodilator drugs before testing. Consult tables 14-4A and B, and review figure 14-4.

Table 14-4A	Selected Pulmonary Function Values for Patient 4			
Name	#	yrs	cm	kg
Patient 4	4	64	174	67.3

Measure, units	Mean	LLN/ULN	Pre-BD	Post-BD
SVC, L	3.89	2.91	3.18	3.92
FVC, L	3.89	2.91	3.09	3.89
IC, L	2.91		2.75	3.31
ERV, L	0.97		0.43	0.61
FRC, L	3.08		4.43	
RV, L	2.11	**2.90**	4.00	
TLC, L (LLN)	5.99	4.79	7.18	
TLC, L (**ULN**)	5.99	**7.19**	7.18	
RV/TLC	0.35	**0.44**	0.56	
FEV$_1$, L	2.98	2.17	1.65	2.01
FEV$_3$, L	3.48	2.58	2.44	2.90
%FEV$_1$/FVC	76.6	67.2	53.4%	
%FEV$_3$/FVC	89.6	84.6	79.0%	
MVV, L/min	119	86	49	
SBO$_2$ ^%N$_2$/L (**ULN**)		**2.6**	9.1	
IVC, L			2.75	
VA', L	5.99		5.20	
VA'/TLC	0.95	>0.85	0.72	
DLCO, mL/min/torr	27.4	20.5	6.7	
DLCO/VA'	4.57	3.43	1.29	

Table 14-4B	Values for 3 Trials Pre- and Post-BD	
%FEV₁/FVC	Pre-BD	Post-BD
Trial 1	51	50
Trial 2	54	50
Trial 3	51	52
t-test $p =$		0.165
Rank order $p =$		NS
$FEF_{25-75\%}$		
Trial 1	0.60	0.56
Trial 2	0.71	0.61
Trial 3	0.57	0.72
t-test $p =$		0.480
Rank order $p =$		NS
FEV_1		
Trial 1	1.47	1.93
Trial 2	1.65	1.93
Trial 3	1.54	2.01
t-test $p =$		0.001
Rank order $p =$		0.05
FEV_3		
Trial 1	2.21	2.79
Trial 2	2.44	2.62
Trial 3	2.26	2.90
t-test $p =$		0.006
Rank order $p =$		0.05

Question 14-4-1: Why is the VA'/TLC low?

Answer: Maldistribution of ventilation. During the 10 seconds breath holding period of the DLCO measurement, the inert gas methane reached only 5.2 L of the patient's TLC of 7.2 L, despite the fact that the patient's inspiratory volume during the maneuver equaled his forced vital capacity. He also has maldistribution of ventilation by the single breath O_2 test.

Question 14-4-2: What is your diagnosis? Does this entire test fit asthma or bronchitis or emphysema?

Answer: The low DLCO/VA' is typical of emphysema and not asthma. The patient's symptoms indicate that he also has chronic bronchitis.

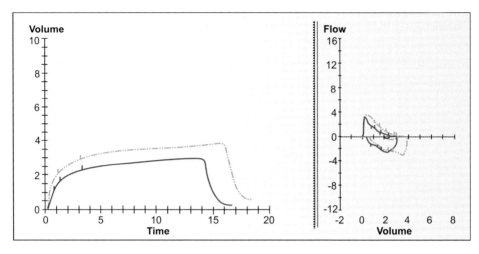

Figure 14-4 The volume-time tracings are on the left; the flow-volume tracings are on the right. The best pre-BD tracings are solid lines; the best post-BD tracings are dotted lines.

Case 14-5

This is a case of 59-year-old black woman, who has had systemic sclerosis for several years but has had no lung function tests before. She complains of fatigue. Note figure 14-5 and table 14-5.

Comment: The patient cooperated well but had difficulty with the MVV maneuver because of the pain. In normal individuals and patients with obstructive lung disease, the MVV in L/min usually approximates 40 times the FEV_1 in liters. Review the flow-volume tracing and the data in table 14-5.

Table 14-5	Selected Pulmonary Function Values for Patient 5			
Name	#	yrs	cm	Kg
Patient 5	5	59	163	54
Measure, units	Mean		LLN/ULN	Actual
SVC, L	2.89		2.19	1.28
FVC, L	2.89		2.19	1.40
IC, L	2.17			0.88
ERV, L	0.72			0.52
FRC, L	2.41			2.33
RV, L	1.68		**2.29**	1.81
TLC, L (LLN)	4.57		3.66	3.21
TLC, L (**ULN**)	4.57		**5.49**	3.21
RV/TLC	0.37		**0.46**	0.56
FEV_1, L	2.27		1.70	1.19
FEV_3, L	2.65		2.00	1.39
%FEV_1/FVC	78.6		69.1	85.0%
%FEV_3/FVC	91.5		87.0	99.3%
MVV, L/min	91		66	27
SBO_2 ^%N_2/L (**ULN**)			**5.7**	3.2
IVC, L				1.20
VA', L	4.57			2.50
VA'/TLC	0.95		>0.85	0.78
DLCO, mL/min/torr	20.5		15.4	5.5
DLCO/VA'	4.49		3.36	2.20

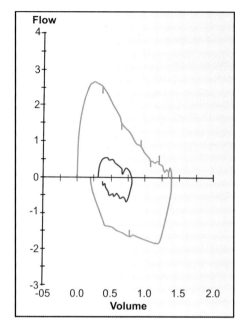

Figure 14-5 Flow-volume tracing. Note the volume scale

Question 14-5-1: Is her FEV$_1$ reduced because of obstructive airway disease?

Answer: No, the FEV$_1$ is reduced because the FVC and TLC are reduced. She has restrictive, not obstructive lung disease. The FEV$_1$/FVC ratio is above average, probably due to increased lung elastic recoil. In interstitial disease, which she has, one often finds the measured MVV increased 50 to 60 times the measured FEV$_1$. In this case pain and/or weakness prevented her from having a higher MVV.

Question 14-5-2: What do the low VA'/TLC, low VA', low DLCO/VA' and very low DLCO indicate in this patient?

Answer: Low VA'/TLC indicates mild maldistribution of ventilation; low VA' indicates restrictive lung disease; low DLCO/VA' indicates low volume of pulmonary capillaries in the ventilated lung; low DLCO indicated very low overall volume of pulmonary capillaries, no doubt due to their destruction by the interstitial lung disease.

Question 14-5-3: Should pulmonary function tests be obtained in all individuals with systemic sclerosis, dermatomyositis, systemic lupus erythematosus (SLE) and similar diseases?

Answer: Yes, since lung disease may be asymptomatic because of other organ diseases and is so often undetected. In systemic sclerosis, lung disease can be serious and lethal.

Case 14-6

This is a case of 47-year-old Asian male with a 45 year-pack history of cigarette smoking. This individual complains of mild dyspnea without cough, sputum or wheezing. He is also a heavy consumer of alcoholic beverages and has lost 10 pounds of weight in the last few months. Note table 14-6 and figures 14-6A and B. Look at spirometric data only, and figure 14-6A before answering question 1.

Table 14-6	Selected Pulmonary Function Values for Patient 6			
Name	#	yrs	cm	Kg
Patient 6	6	47	167	53
Measure, units	Mean		LLN/ULN	Actual
SVC, L	3.87		2.90	4.39
FVC, L	3.87		2.90	4.50
IC, L	2.90			2.38
ERV, L	0.97			2.12
FRC, L	2.64			3.98
RV, L	1.67		**2.46**	1.86
TLC, L (LLN)	5.54		4.43	6.36
TLC, L (**ULN**)	5.54		**6.65**	6.36
RV/TLC	0.30		**0.39**	0.29
FEV_1, L	3.13		2.32	3.56
FEV_3, L	3.61		2.70	4.37
%FEV_1/FVC	81.0		71.5	79.1%
%FEV_3/FVC	93.1		88.1	97.1%
MVV, L/min	125		92	134
SBO_2 ^%N_2/L (**ULN**)			**1.8**	2.6
IVC, L				4.10
VA', L	5.54			6.30
VA'/TLC	0.95		>0.85	0.99
DLCO, mL/min/torr	28.9		21.7	19.3
DLCO/VA'	5.22		3.91	3.06

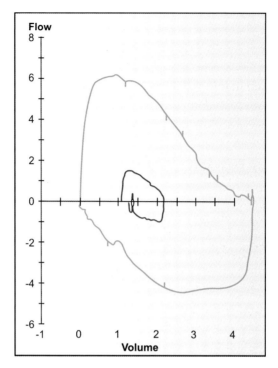

Figure 14-6A Flow-volume tracing

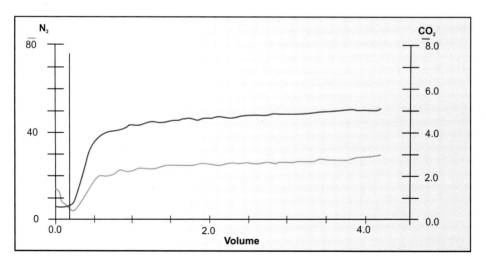

Figure 14-6B Single breath oxygen test tracings. Full inhalation of O_2 followed by slow exhalation. The percent nitrogen of exhalate (lower blue tracing) is scaled on the left Y-axis; the percent CO_2 of exhalate (higher red tracing) is scaled on the right Y-axis.

Question 14-6-1: Look at spirometry only. What diagnosis do you favor? Consider the opinion of a recent editorial summarizing the recommendation statement of US Preventive Task Force; screening for chronic obstructive pulmonary disease using spirometry; published in the 2008 *Annals of Internal Medicine*, volume 148, pages 529 to 534 which state, "Only if both the FEV_1/FVC ratio and the FEV_1 value are below the LLN after effective therapy for airway disease – and only in patients who have smoked more than 20 years – is it plausible to associate smoking with harm done to the lung."

Answer: If you consider the last statement only you would opine that the patient does not have any damaged lung from smoking and therefore, certainly could not have chronic obstructive pulmonary disease. But please continue further.

Question 14-6-2: What is your diagnosis after looking at the entire test?

Answer: It should be emphysema. The low DLCO, and especially the low DLCO/VA' strongly favor this diagnosis. This is not maldistribution of ventilation since the VA'/TLC ratio is normal. He has lost pulmonary capillary volume. In part because his lung volume is high and near the ULN, the FEV_1/FVC is just below the predicted mean and is not near or below the LLN.

Question 14-6-3: In addition to a low FEV_1/FVC, some authorities require that the measured FEV_1 be below the LLN. How can one identify this study as obstructive airways disease when his FEV_1 is above 80% of mean predicted?

Answer: Authoritative opinions are sometimes incorrect. Consider that there is much variability in absolute values of FEV_1, FEV_3, FEV_6, FVC, and TLC values in individuals of the same gender, height, age and ethnicity. Therefore, it is not reasonable to exclude airways disease on the basis of any absolute FEV_1 value. His physician, before obtaining his pulmonary function test, had obtained a high resolution chest scan. The scan showed no evidence of malignancy, but multiple areas of mild to moderate emphysema were clearly visible.

Case 14-7

For several months this 42-year-old Latin male has experienced moderate shortness of breath, and some wheezing and hoarseness, but had no cough or sputum. He had no known exposure to toxic dusts or fumes except for 3 pack-years of smoking a decade ago. He had not received any therapy. There was no swelling of the neck. Note figure 14-7 and tables 14-7A and B.

Table 14-7A	Selected Pulmonary Function Values for Patient 7			
Name	#	yrs	cm	kg
Patient 7	7	42	170	85.5

Measure, units	Mean		LLN/ULN	Actual
SVC, L	4.16		3.19	4.63
FVC, L	4.16		3.19	4.87
IC, L	3.12			4.03
ERV, L	1.04			0.74
FRC, L	2.66			2.83
RV, L	1.62		**2.42**	2.09
TLC, L (LLN)	5.79		4.63	6.96
TLC, L (**ULN**)	5.79		**6.94**	6.96
RV/TLC	0.28		**0.37**	0.30
FEV_1, L	3.38		2.57	3.33
FEV_3, L	3.91		3.01	4.74
%FEV_1/FVC	81.3		71.8	68.4%
%FEV_3/FVC	93.9		88.9	97.3%
MVV, L/min	135		102	64
SBO_2 ^%N_2/L (**ULN**)			**1.6**	1.4
IVC, L				4.50
VA', L	5.79			6.40
VA'/TLC	0.95		>0.85	0.92
DLCO, mL/min/torr	30.8		23.1	38.6
DLCO/VA'	5.32		3.99	6.03

Table 14-7B	Values for 3 Trials Pre-BD and Post- BD	
FEV$_1$	Pre-BD	Post-BD
Trial 1	2.76	3.95
Trial 2	3.33	4.12
Trial 3	3.06	4.04
t-test p=		0.002
Rank order p=		0.05
FEV$_3$		
Trial 1	4.67	4.75
Trial 2	4.65	4.78
Trial 3	4.74	4.83
t-test p=		0.025
Rank order p=		0.05
FEV$_6$		
Trial 1	4.85	4.89
Trial 2	4.85	4.95
Trial 3	4.81	4.99
t-test p=		0.014
Rank order p=		0.05
Pk Insp Flow		
Trial 1	3.38	4.65
Trial 2	2.46	4.97
Trial 3	3.96	4.06
t-test p=		0.032
Rank order p =		0.05

Question 14-7-1: Look at the flow-volume tracing and the time-volume tracing in figure 14-6A. What pattern do they show?

Answer: They both show the same pattern, that of larger airway obstruction with reduced peak inspiratory and expiratory flow. In the flow volume tracing the early and mid-expiration constant flow is displayed as a horizontal line and as a reduced constant flow during mid-inspiration. On the time-volume display, the linear diagonal lines also display nearly constant flows. At end exhalation, the flow rate becomes lower as smaller airways rather than larger airways now inhibit flow.

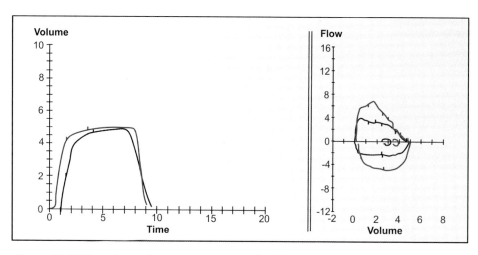

Figure 14-7 The volume-time tracings are on the left; the flow-volume tracings are on the right. The best pre-BD tracings are black lines and the best post-BD tracings are red lines.

Question 14-7-2: Exactly where is the larger airway obstruction anatomically located? **Answer:** Not sure, but much more likely to be in the pharynx or larynx or extra-thoracic trachea. The ratio of FEV_3/FVC of 4.74/4.87 or 97.3% indicates that there is very little or no obstruction of the latest emptying airways or airspaces. Such a finding would be very unusual for asthma.

Question 14-7-3: Why are the DLCO and DLCO/VA' higher than average? **Answer:** The pulmonary capillaries have a higher than average volume. Elevated DLCO is often seen in asthma. It is unclear why it is elevated in this patient.

Question 14-7-4: Look at the spirometry values before and after four breaths of aerosolized albuterol in table 14-7B. Is the result astonishing? **Answer:** The variability of flow before and after aerosolized albuterol is surprising as is the striking improvement in flow after albuterol. Both inspiratory and expiratory flow are markedly improved. The invariable high ratio of FEV_3/FEV_6 in all of the forced exhalations would also be very unusual in asthma. Laryngoscopy should be helpful.

Case 14-8

This 55-year-old woman, a heavy smoker in the past, thought that she had asthma. Note tables 14-8A and B, and figure 14-8.

Table 14-8A	Selected Pulmonary Function Values for Patient 8			
Name	#	yrs	cm	kg
Patient 8	8	55	168	97

Measure, units	Mean		LLN/**ULN**	Pre-BD	Post-BD
SVC, L	3.18		2.47	2.73	2.94
FVC, L	3.18		2.47	2.82	2.94
IC, L	2.38			2.58	2.76
ERV, L	0.79			0.15	0.16
FRC, L	2.50			2.12	
RV, L	1.71		**2.32**	1.97	
TLC, L (LLN)	4.88		3.91	4.70	
TLC, L **(ULN)**	4.88		**5.86**	4.70	
RV/TLC	0.35		**0.44**	0.42	
FEV_1, L	2.51		1.94	1.98	2.11
FEV_3, L	2.93		2.28	2.47	2.61
%FEV_1/FVC	79.0		69.6	70.2%	
%FEV_3/FVC	92.2		87.7	87.6%	
MVV, L/min	100		76	93	96
SBO_2 ^%N_2/L **(ULN)**			**2.8**	4.00	
IVC, L				2.80	
VA', L	4.88			4.30	
VA'/TLC	0.95		>0.85	0.91	
DLCO, mL/min/torr	22.0		16.5	13.4	
DLCO/VA'	4.51		3.38	3.12	

Table 14-8B	Values for 3 Trials Pre-BD and Post- BD	
FEV$_1$	Pre-BD	Post-BD
Trial 1	1.98	2.09
Trial 2	1.98	2.07
Trial 3	2.01	2.11
t-test p=		0.001
Rank order p=		0.05
FEV$_3$		
Trial 1	2.44	2.52
Trial 2	2.47	2.53
Trial 3	2.49	2.61
t-test p=		0.027
Rank order p=		0.05
FEV$_6$		
Trial 1	2.66	2.73
Trial 2	2.68	2.73
Trial 3	2.70	2.80
t-test p=		0.024
Rank order p=		0.05
FVC		
Trial 1	2.83	2.94
Trial 2	2.82	2.88
Trial 3	2.81	2.94
t-test p=		0.004
Rank order p =		0.05

Question 14-8-1: Look at the flow-volume tracing before the patient received aerosolized albuterol. For a 55-year-old woman, does this appear to be airway obstruction? Does it also look like obesity?

Answer: Yes, it does appears to be an airway obstruction and a case of obesity as is evident from concave tracing during forced exhalation and very low ERV.

Question 14-8-2: Compare the predicted and pre-BD and post-BD values for spirometry and lung volumes in table 14-8. Are the VC, RV, TLC, RV/TLC, FEV$_1$, FEV$_3$, %FEV$_1$/FVC, or %FEV$_3$/FVC outside of 95% confidence limits?

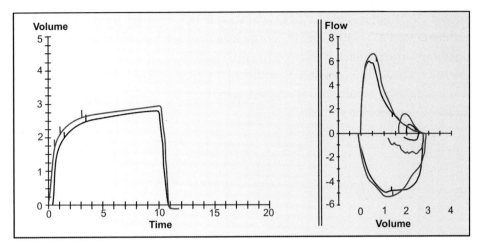

Figure 14-8 The volume-time tracings are on the left; the flow-volume tracings are on the right. The best pre-BD tracings are black lines; the best post-BD tracings are red lines.

Answer: No, consider the opinion of a recent editorial in the *Primary Care Respiratory Journal* (Britain) summarizing the recommendation statement of US Preventive Task Force. Screening for chronic obstructive pulmonary disease using spirometry, published in the 2008 *Annals of Internal Medicine*, volume 148, pages 529 to 534. The editorial states, "Only if both the FEV_1/FVC ratio and the FEV_1 value are below the LLN after effective therapy for airway disease – and only in patients who have smoked more than 20 years – is it plausible to associate smoking with harm done to the lung." But please continue further.

Question 14-8-3: Note the gas transfer (DLCO) measurements. Because the IVC was over 90% of the baseline VC and the VA'/TLC was normal, there was no evidence of maldistribution of ventilation on the single-breath test. The DLCO and DLCO/VA' are significantly decreased, indicating loss of pulmonary capillary bed. Are these gas transfer measurements compatible with asthma or emphysema?

Answer: These measurements are compatible with emphysema, but not asthma.

Question 14-8-4: Considering the findings in this patient, do you consider the opinions of the editorial, which summarizes the Task Force, binding on your interpretations.

Answer: No, the opinions of the editorial, summarizing the Task Force are not binding with our interpretations.

Question 14-8-5: Now please review table 14-8B, which shows details of the pre-BD and post-BD tests. Do any of these values meet the requirements of the ATS/ERS guidelines which require both an increase of 200 mL and an increase in 12% of the FEV_1 or FVC to identify a positive bronchodilator response.

Answer: No, neither the FEV_1, FEV_3, FEV_6, nor FVC changes meet those criteria. Yet the FEV_1, FEV_3, FEV_6, and FVC responses are each consistent and statistically significant. The changes average between 4% and 5%.

Question 14-8-6: Is it possible that the ATS/ERS guideline criteria are also unreasonable? How would you report these tests?

Answer: Your decision to make.

Case 14-9

This 45-year-old black woman was hospitalized with severe shortness of breath. She had never smoked and did not have cough or sputum. She had cardiomegaly, and pericardial and pleural effusions. Note table 14-9 and figures 14-9A and B.

Table 14-9	Selected Pulmonary Function Values for Patient 9			
Name	#	yrs	cm	kg
Patient 9	9	45	160	68

Measure, units	Mean		LLN/ULN	Actual
SVC, L	3.01		2.31	1.03
FVC, L	3.01		2.31	1.01
IC, L	2.26			0.68
ERV, L	0.75			0.35
FRC, L	2.17			1.06
RV, L	1.42		**2.03**	0.74
TLC, L (LLN)	4.43		3.55	1.77
TLC, L (**ULN**)	4.43		**5.32**	
RV/TLC	0.32		**0.41**	0.42
FEV_1, L	2.48		1.91	0.81
FEV_3, L	2.85		2.20	0.98
%FEV_1/FVC	82.4		72.9	80.2%
%FEV_3/FVC	94.4		89.9	97.0%
MVV, L/min	99		75	39
SBO_2 ^%N_2/L (**ULN**)			7.9	
IVC, L				0.91
VA', L	4.43			1.79
VA'/TLC	0.95		>0.85	1.01
DLCO, mL/min/torr	21.8		16.3	8.5
DLCO/VA'	4.91		3.68	4.75

Question 14-9-1: Note the very low FEV$_1$ and FEV$_3$. Does this patient have evidence of obstructive lung disease?

Answer: Although the FEV$_1$ and FEV$_3$ are very low, the FVC and TLC are also very low, while the FEV$_1$/FVC and FEV$_3$/FVC are normal. She does not have obstructive lung disease.

Question 14-9-2: Does she have restrictive lung disease?

Answer: She has severe lung restriction. If we consider her known pleural effusion as evidence of lung disease, she has severe restrictive lung disease. Her restriction is also caused by her cardiomegaly and pericardial effusion.

Question 14-9-3: Why is the DLCO/VA' normal?

Answer: It is doubtful that she has any intrinsic lung disease as the ventilated lung appears to be adequately perfused. The loss in DLCO appears to be parallel to her loss of lung volume. Sometimes with heart failure the DLCO/VA' is increased due to congestion of the pulmonary capillaries; sometimes with heart failure the DLCO/VA' is decreased due to pulmonary edema.

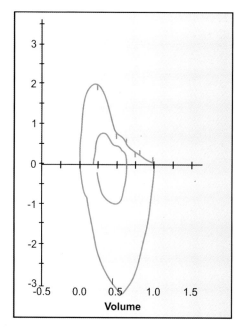

Figure 14-9A Flow-volume tracing. Note the volume scale.

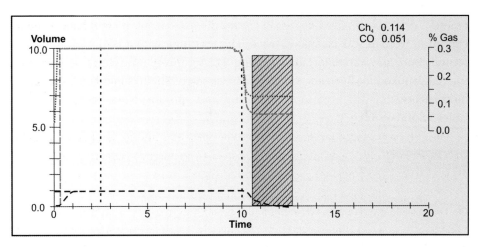

Figure 14-9B Single breath gas transfer or diffusing capacity test. Time is on the X-axis. The left Y-axis is volume. The lowest tracing shows the IVC, held for 10 seconds followed by the forced exhalation. The right Y-axis shows the concentrations of methane (upper tracing) and CO (lower tracing) in the exhalate, measured during the time with oblique hatching.

Case 14-10

This adult woman was evaluated twice. The first time with a BMI of 33.4 and the second time, 2.5 years later, after gaining 34.5 kg more, now with a BMI of 46.9. She had smoked for 31 years, stopping 14 years ago. She has become increasingly short of breath, with occasional wheezing and sputum. Note figure 14-10 and tables 14-10A and B.

Table 14-10A Selected Pulmonary Function Values for Patient 10 (Test 2.5 years Ago)					
Name	#	yrs	cm	kg	date
Patient 10	10	60	160	85.5	2.5 years ago

Measure, units	Mean	LLN/**ULN**	Pre-BD	Post-BD
SVC, L	3.08	2.38	2.31	2.39
FVC, L	3.08	2.38	2.17	2.13
IC, L	2.31		2.19	2.28
ERV, L	0.77		0.12	0.11
FRC, L	2.62		2.81	
RV, L	1.85	**2.46**	2.69	
TLC, L (LLN)	4.93	3.95	5.00	
TLC, L (**ULN**)	4.93	**5.92**	5.00	
RV/TLC	0.37	**0.47**	0.54	
FEV_1, L	2.40	1.83	1.45	1.50
FEV_3, L	2.82	2.17	1.89	1.92
%FEV_1/FVC	77.8	68.3	66.8%	
%FEV_3/FVC	91.3	86.8	87.1%	
MVV, L/min	96	71	69	67
SBO_2 ^%N_2/L (**ULN**)		**3.7**	6.5	
IVC, L			2.30	
VA', L	4.93		4.00	
VA'/TLC	0.95	>0.85	0.80	
DLCO, mL/min/torr	20.8	15.6	11.7	
DLCO/VA'	4.22	3.17	2.93	

SpO_2 = 93%

Table 14-10B	Selected Pulmonary Function Values for Patient 10 (Current/Second Test)				
Name	#	yrs	cm	Kg	Date
Patient 10	10	63	160	120	Current

Measure, units	Mean		LLN/ULN	Pre-BD	Post-BD
SVC, L	3.02		2.32	2.09	2.35
FVC, L	3.02		2.32	2.12	2.39
IC, L	2.27			1.87	2.15
ERV, L	0.76			0.25	0.20
FRC, L	2.66			2.35	
RV, L	1.90		**2.51**	2.10	
TLC, L (LLN)	4.92		3.94	4.22	
TLC, L (**ULN**)	4.92		**5.91**	4.22	
RV/TLC	0.39		**0.48**	0.50	
FEV_1, L	2.33		1.76	1.38	1.63
FEV_3, L	2.74		2.09	1.78	2.08
%FEV_1/FVC	77.0		67.5	65.1%	
%FEV_3/FVC	90.6		86.1	84.0%	
MVV, L/min	93		68	65	72
SBO_2 ^%N_2/L (**ULN**)			**3.8**	7.3	
IVC, L				2.00	
VA', L	4.92			3.20	
VA'/TLC	0.95		>0.85	0.76	
DLCO, mL/min/torr	20.4		15.3	10.0	
DLCO/VA'	4.15		3.11	3.13	

SpO_2 92%

Question 14-10-1: Check table 14-10A. Does this patient have obstructive airways disease?

Answer: Yes, reduced FEV_1/FVC, FEV_1, and elevated RV/TLC show the occurrence of obstructive airways disease.

Question 14-10-2: What else can you figure out from table 14-10A?

Answer: High IC/ERV ratio is the result of her obesity. The resting position of the diaphragm is very high, as the patient has only 0.12 L to further exhale from the

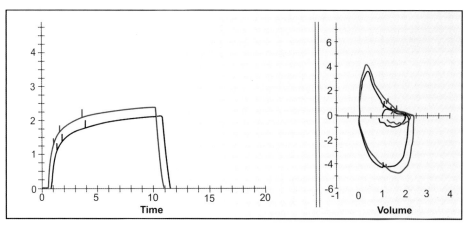

Figure 14-10 The volume-time tracings are on the left; the flow-volume tracings are on the right. The best pre-BD tracings are black lines; the best post-BD tracings are red lines.

resting position of the diaphragm. The DLCO/VA' is low rather than high. Increased DLCO/VA' frequently occurs with obesity and often with asthma. Thus, emphysema seems more likely than asthma. Maldistribution of ventilation is evidenced by low VA' and low VA'/TLC and high SBO_2.

Comment: Weight has increased markedly over two and a half years, yet FVC, IC, and DLCO have decreased only slightly. The RV, TLC, and VA' have decreased a bit more, evidence of compression or restriction of the lung. Note the positive bronchodilator effect now evident.

Question 14-10-3: If she has emphysema, why is not the TLC elevated?

Answer: The TLC is not elevated probably because her severe obesity compresses her thorax. The RV and RV/TLC were both increased on her first test. Only the RV/TLC is increased now.

Question 14-10-4: Could she be in a state of heart failure?

Answer: Yes.

15 Quality Control and Normal Laboratory Variability

INTRODUCTION

In addition to the usual quality control of all laboratory instrumentation there are good reasons to record and evaluate serial pulmonary function tests of one or more laboratory personnel. Such a practice allows one to compare differing pieces of equipment that measure the same variables. It is helpful to evaluate the mean values and natural variability of specific measurements on the same individual on the same equipment over time; and to identify when equipment becomes faulty.

SINGLE EQUIPMENT

Figures 15-1 to 15-3 show serial measurements over a period of time on a single individual using one set of equipment. Note that in figure 15-1, the absolute spirometric values of FVC, FEV_1 and FEV_3 all have higher variability than the ratios of FEV_1/FVC and FEV_3/FVC. The decline in absolute values during month 12, suggests a mild illness or equipment malfunction or problem with calibration. Recall, however,

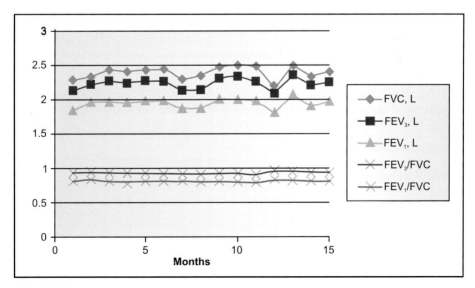

Figure 15-1 Serial spirometric measurements of a single individual at monthly intervals.

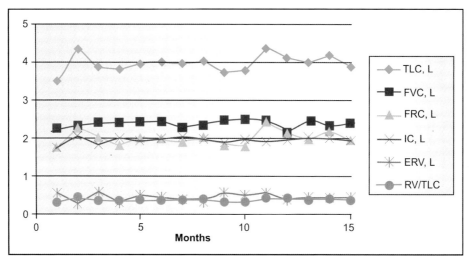

Figure 15-2 Serial lung volume measurments of a single individual at monthly intervals. Values combine spirometric and body plethysmographic measurements. Note higher variability in FRC and TLC than FVC.

that with calibration of most spirometric equipment a 3% difference in volumes is acceptable.

Figure 15-2 adds the body plethysmographic measures to the spirometric values. This graph shows the relative stability of FVC while the IC and ERV are more variable. This leads to greater variability of the RV, FRC and TLC than the FVC.

Figure 15-3 shows that in this cooperative subject, IVC volumes are always very close to FVC volumes of the same day resulting in excellent stability of the DLCO, VA', and DLCO/VA' over the course of an year.

Thus, the changes from one test to another a month apart should be greater than these within a few minutes of each other when judging whether there was significant improvement or deterioration in a patient. When the comparisons are between different laboratories or technicians or different sets of equipment, even greater differences inevitably occur.

COMPARING EQUIPMENT

Table 15-1 compares two sets of equipment from the same manufacturer. One set measures FRC by body plethysmograph, the other by nitrogen washout. This table also allows one to see several things:

1. The relatively high percentage variability of the ERV and IC in both sets of equipment.

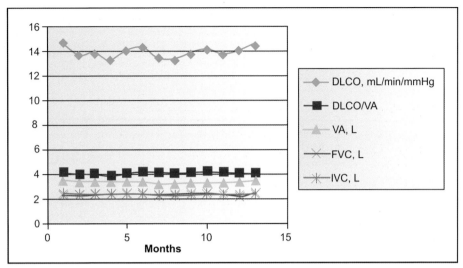

Figure 15-3 Serial gas transfer (DLCO) and allied measurements of a single individual at monthly intervals. At each time, values are the averages of two maneuvers. Note that IVC values are quite similar to separately measured FVC values.

2. The considerable variability of the FRC and TLC measurements (SD for each approximates 200 mL).
3. The high reproducibility of the FEV_1, FEV_3, FVC, and SVC with each method. (The mean differences in the FEV_1 between methods is 38 mL.)
4. The consistent 1% differences in FEV_1/FVC between the two sets of equipment.
5. The high variability of the $FEF_{25-75\%}$ on both sets of equipment (which is not a surprise) compared to other spirometric measures.
6. The relatively high reproducibility of the IVC, DLCO, and DLCO/VA' between the two sets of equipment, with the single breath VA' slightly less variable than the TLC measured by plethysmography or nitrogen washout.

Thus, there can be measurable differences between sets of equipment in the same laboratory.

CONCLUSION

The collection of serial data of one or more laboratory personnel on a continuing basis gives observers appreciation of the natural variability seen in a single laboratory. When data are plotted serially, deviations should be detectable and investigated. When new equipment is added to a laboratory, the comparison of the same individual on older and newer sets of equipment is strongly recommended.

Table 15-1 Comparison of Serial Pulmonary Function Tests of the Same Individual for 15 months on Two Sets of Equipment.

Measure	Spirometer # 1 with Body plethysmograph			Spirometer # 2 with Nitrogen washout			Differences	
	Mean	SD	COV,%	Mean	SD	COV,%	Absolute	Percent
SVC, L	2.391	0.070	2.9%	2.377	0.070	2.9%	0.015	0.6%
FVC, L	2.395	0.095	4.0%	2.380	0.083	3.5%	0.015	0.6%
IC, L	1.958	0.082	4.2%	1.836	0.110	6.0%	0.122	6.2%
ERV, L	0.462	0.100	21.7%	0.528	0.115	21.7%	0.066	14.3%
FRC, L	2.017	0.189	9.4%	1.918	0.234	12.2%	0.099	4.9%
RV, L	1.549	0.229	14.8%	1.356	0.224	16.5%	0.193	12.4%
TLC, L	3.975	0.221	5.6%	3.737	0.236	6.3%	0.238	6.0%
RV/TLC	0.388	0.037	9.5%	0.361	0.038	10.5%	0.027	6.9%
FEV_1, L	1.953	0.070	3.6%	1.915	0.055	2.9%	0.038	1.9%
FEV_3, L	2.233	0.080	3.6%	2.188	0.071	3.2%	0.045	2.0%
FEV_1/FVC	0.816	0.013	1.6%	0.805	0.016	1.9%	0.011	1.3%
FEV_3/FVC	0.933	0.014	1.5%	0.920	0.016	1.7%	0.013	1.4%
$FEF_{25-75\%}$, L/s	2.151	0.175	8.1%	2.019	0.208	10.3%	0.132	6.1%
IVC, L	2.35	0.092	3.9%	2.32	0.126	5.5%	0.033	1.4%
VA', L	3.33	0.150	4.5%	3.47	0.191	5.5%	0.14	4.0%
DLCO, unit	13.71	0.719	5.2%	13.87	0.720	5.2%	0.16	1.2%
DLCO/VA'	4.11	0.095	2.3%	4.01	0.141	3.5%	0.11	2.6%

Appendix A
Recommended Reference Equations for Pulmonary Function Tests

There are many different reference equations available for predicting normal values. These in Appendix A have been selected because they yield approximate mean or near mean values of series of apparently normal subjects. The "white" or "W" equations should be used for European, Australian, and American individuals (including Latins) who do not consider themselves "black". The "majority" or "M" equations should be used for Asian, African, Polynesian individuals, as well as those who consider themselves "black."

In all equations, volumes are in L, flows in L/time, ages in years, heights in centimeters, weights in kg DLCO in mL/min/L, SBO_2 is in percentage change in N_2/L of known measured VC, and ratios are in fractions or percentages. For both genders and all ethnicities **for ages of 20–24 years, substitute age 25** in equations for SVC, FVC, FEV_1, FEV_3, FEV_6, IC, ERV, FRC, RV, TLC,VA', and DLCO. Mean and RSD (or Syx or SEE) values are given. For spirometric volumes and flows multiply the RSD values by 1.645 and subtract from mean values to find 95% confidence limits of lower limits of normal (LLN). For TLC and RV, upper limit of normal (ULN) values are also useful. For TLC and DLCO equations LLN or ULN are given directly as 75% or 125% or 80% or 120%, respectively, of mean predicted values. For some volumes no 95% confidence limits are given.

1. "White" or "W" Adult Women; Predicted Mean and Variability
- FVC or SVC, $L = -3.387 - 0.0201 \times yrs + 0.04798 \times cm$; RSD = 0.427
- FEV_1, $L = -1.568 - 0.0239 \times yrs + 0.03376 \times cm$; RSD = 0.346
- FEV_3, $L = -2.614 - 0.02537 \times yrs + 0.043454 \times cm$; RSD = 0.393
- FEV_6, $L = -3.044 - 0.023 \times yrs + 0.0462 \times cm$; RSD = 0.413
- Peak expiratory flow, mid expiratory flow, peak inspiratory flow, L/sec = look at tracings
- MVV, L/min = $FEV_1 \times 40$, RSD = 15
- %FEV_1/FVC (Use FVC equation value divided into FEV_1 equation value). RSD = 5.77%
- %FEV_1/FEV_6 (Use FEV_6 equation value divided into FEV_1 equation value). RSD = 3.62%
- %FEV_3/FVC (Use FVC equation value divided into FEV_3 equation value). RSD = 2.76%
- %FEV_3/FEV_6 (Use FEV_6 equation value divided into FEV_3 equation value). RSD = 1.96%

- IC/ERV = 1.1+ 0.03 × years
- IC = VC x (1.1 + 0.03 × years)/(2.1 + 0.03 × years)
- ERV = VC – IC
- RV, L = –2.258 + 0.017 x yrs + 0.0193 x cm; RSD = 0.370
- FRC, L = ERV + RV
- TLC, = FVC + RV, or = –5.545 + 0.06533 x cm (values differ minimally) LLN:ULN = 80:120%
- RV/TLC (Use RV value divided by TLC value); RSD = 0.051
- VA' = predicted mean TLC value
- VA'/TLC = actual single breath VA' value divided by actual TLC value: normal ≥ 0.85
- DLCO = –4.34 – 0.139 x yrs + 0.20944 x cm; LLN:ULN = 75:125%
- DLCO/VA' – predicted DLCO/predicted VA'; LLN:ULN = 75:125%
- SBO_2, %ΔN_2/L: ULN = 8.0/ actual FVC (note, use %ΔN_2 per L not, per 500 mL).

2. "Majority" or "M" Adult Women; Predicted Mean and Variability

- FVC or SVC, L = 0.89 × (–3.387 – 0.0201 × yrs + 0.04798 × cm); RSD = 0.427
- FEV_1, L = 0.90 × (–1.568 – 0.0239 × yrs + 0.03376 × cm); RSD = 0.346
- FEV_3, L = 0.89 × (–2.614 – 0.02537 × yrs + 0.043454 × cm); RSD = 0.393
- FEV_6, L = 0.89 × (–3.044 – 0.023 × yrs + 0.0462 × cm); RSD = 0.413
- Peak expiratory flow, mid expiratory flow, peak inspiratory flow, L/sec = look at tracings
- MVV, L/min = FEV_1 x 40, RSD = 15
- %FEV_1/FVC (Use FVC equation value divided into FEV_1 equation value). RSD = 5.77%
- %FEV_1/FEV_6 (Use FEV_6 equation value divided into FEV_1 equation value). RSD = 3.62%
- %FEV_3/FVC (Use FVC equation value divided into FEV_3 equation value). RSD = 2.76%
- %FEV_3/FEV_6 (Use FEV_6 equation value divided into FEV_3 equation value). RSD = 1.96%
- IC/ERV = 1.1 + 0.03 × years
- IC = VC × (1.1 + 0.03 × years)/(2.1 + 0.03 × years)
- ERV = VC – IC
- RV = 0.89 x (–2.258 + 0.017 x yrs + 0.0193 x cm); RSD = 0.370
- FRC, L = ERV + RV
- TLC, L = FVC + RV, or = 0.89 x (–5.545 + 0.06533 x cm (values differ minimally) LLN:ULN = 80:120%
- RV/TLC (Use RV value divided by TLC value); RSD = 0.051
- VA' = predicted mean TLC value

- VA'/TLC = actual single breath VA' value divided by actual TLC value: normal ≥ 0.85
- DLCO = 0.95 x (= −4.34 − 0.139 x yrs + 0.20944 x cm); LLN:ULN = 75:125%
- DLCO/VA' = predicted DLCO/predicted VA'; LLN:ULN = 75:125%
- SBO_2, $\%\Delta N_2/L$: ULN = 8.0/ actual FVC (note, use $\%\Delta N_2$ per L not, per 500 mL).

3. "White" or "W" Adult Men; Predicted Mean and Variability

- FVC or SVC, L = −5.396 − 0.0261 x yrs + 0.0657 x cm; RSD = 0.591
- FEV_1, L = −2.639 − 0.0286 × yrs + 0.0447 × cm; RSD = 0.493
- FEV_3, L = −4.362 − 0.0327 × yrs + 0.05958 × cm; RSD = 0.548
- FEV_6, L = −4.889 − 0.0301 × yrs + 0.0631 × cm; RSD = 0.566
- Peak expiratory flow, mid expiratory flow, peak inspiratory flow, L/sec = look at tracings
- MVV, L/min = FEV_1 × 40, RSD = 20
- $\%FEV_1/FVC$ (Use FVC equation value divided into FEV_1 equation value). RSD = 5.75%
- $\%FEV_1/FEV_6$ (Use FEV_6 equation value divided into FEV_1 equation value). RSD = 5.05%
- $\%FEV_3/FVC$ (Use FVC equation value divided into FEV_3 equation value). RSD = 3.06%
- $\%FEV_3/FEV_6$ (Use FEV_6 equation value divided into FEV_3 equation value). RSD = 1.49%
- IC/ERV = 1.1+ 0.03 × years
- IC = VC × (1.1 + 0.03 × years)/(2.1 + 0.03 × years)
- ERV = VC − IC
- RV, L = −2.164 + 0.0213 × yrs + 0.0182 × cm; RSD = 0.418
- FRC, L = ERV + RV
- TLC, L = FVC + RV, or = −7.624 + 0.083 x cm (values differ minimally) LLN:ULN = 80:120%
- RV/TLC (Use RV value divided by TLC value); RSD = 0.055
- VA' = predicted mean TLC value
- VA'/TLC = actual single breath VA' value divided by actual TLC value: normal ≥ 0.85
- DLCO = −10.06 − 0.22 x yrs + 0.3043 x cm; LLN:ULN = 75:125%
- DLCO/VA' = predicted DLCO/ predicted VA'; LLN:ULN = 75:125%
- SBO_2, $\%\Delta N_2/L$: ULN = 8.0/ actual FVC (note, use $\%\Delta N_2$ per L, not per 500 mL).

4. "Majority" or "M" Adult Men; Predicted Mean and Variability

- FVC or SVC, L = 0.89 (−5.396 − 0.0261 x yrs + 0.0657 x cm); RSD = 0.591
- FEV_1, L = 0.90 x (−2.639 − 0.0286 x yrs + 0.0447 x cm); RSD = 0.493
- FEV_3, L = 0.89 x (−4.362 − 0.0327 x yrs + 0.05958 x cm); RSD = 0.548

- FEV$_6$, L = 0.89 x (−4.889 − 0.0301 x yrs + 0.0631 x cm); RSD = 0.566
- Peak expiratory flow, mid expiratory flow, peak inspiratory flow, L/sec = look at tracings
- MVV, L/min = FEV1 x 40, RSD = 20
- %FEV$_1$/FVC (Use FVC equation value divided into FEV$_1$ equation value). RSD = 5.75%
- %FEV$_1$/FEV6 (Use FEV6 equation value divided into FEV$_1$ equation value). RSD = 5.05%
- %FEV3/FVC (Use FVC equation value divided into FEV$_3$ equation value). RSD = 3.06%
- %FEV3/FEV6 (Use FEV6 equation value divided into FEV$_3$ equation value). RSD = 1.49%
- IC/ERV = 1.1+ 0.03 x years
- IC = VC × (1.1 + 0.03 × years)/(2.1 + 0.03 × years)
- ERV = VC − IC
- RV, L = 0.89 × (−2.164 + 0.0213 × yrs + 0.0182 x cm); RSD = 0.418
- FRC, L = ERV + RV
- TLC, L = FVC + RV, or 0.89 × (−7.624 + 0.083 × cm) (values differ minimally) LLN:ULN = 80:120%
- RV/TLC = (use RV value divided by TLC value); RSD = 0.055
- VA' = predicted mean TLC value
- VA'/TLC = actual single breath VA' value divided by actual TLC value: normal ≥ 0.85
- DLCO = 0.95 x (= −10.06 − 0.22 x yrs + 0.3043 x cm); LLN:ULN = 75:125%
- DLCO/VA' = predicted DLCO/ predicted VA'; LLN:ULN = 75:125%
- SBO$_2$, %ΔN$_2$/L: ULN = 8.0/ actual FVC (note, use %ΔN$_2$ per L, not per 500 mL).

Appendix B
Other Pulmonary Function Reference Equations

The equations, listed by first author and year of publication, are for "white" subjects unless otherwise stated.

1. Billiet L, Baisier W, Naedts JP. Effet de la taille, et du sefe de l'age sur la capacitie de diffusion pulmonaire de l'adult normal. *J Physiol*. 1963;55:199–200.
   Men: DLCO (mL/min/mmHg) = $-54.7 - 0.24 \times$ yrs $+ 0.576 \times$ cm
   Women: DLCO (mL/min/mmHg) = $-5.93 - 0.16 \times$ yrs $+ 0.219 \times$ cm

2. Crapo RO, Morris AH. Standardized single–breath normal values for diffusing capacity. *Am Rev Respir Dis*. 1981;123:185–9.
   Men: DLCO (mL/min/mmHg) = $-26.3 - 0.22 \times$ yrs $+ 0.416 \times$ cm
   Women: DLCO (mL/min/mmHg) = $-11.1 - 0.14 \times$ yrs $+ 0.256 \times$ cm

3. Crapo RO, Morris AH, Gardner RM. Reference spirometric values using techniques and equipment that meet ATS requirements. *Am Rev Respir Dis*. 1981;123:659–64.

   Men
   FVC (L) = $-4.65 - 0.0214 \times$ yrs $+ 0.06 \times$ cm; RSD = 0.644
   FEV_1 (L) = $-2.19 - 0.0244 \times$ yrs $+ 0.0414 \times$ cm; RSD = 0.486
   FEV_3 (L) = $-3.512 - 0.0271 \times$ yrs $+ 0.0535 \times$ cm; RSD = 0.587
   FEV_1/FVC (%) = $+110.49 - 0.152 \times$ yr $- 0.13 \times$ cm; RSD = 4.78
   FEV_3/FVC (%) = $+112.09 - 0.145 \times$ yrs $- 0.0627 \times$ cm; RSD = 2.68
   $FEF_{25-75\%}$ (L/sec) = $+2.133 - 0.0380 \times$ yrs $+ 0.0204 \times$ cm; RSD = 0.962

   Women
   FVC (L) = $-3.59 - 0.0216 \times$ yrs $+ 0.0491 \times$ cm; RSD = 0.393
   FEV_1 (L) = $-1.578 - 0.0255 \times$ yrs $+ 0.0342 \times$ cm; RSD = 0.326
   FEV_3 (L) = $-2.745 - 0.0257 \times$ yrs $+ 0.0442 \times$ cm; RSD = 0.360
   FEV_1/FVC (%) = $+126.58 - 0.252 \times$ yr $- 0.202 \times$ cm; RSD = 5.26
   FEV_3/FVC (%) = $+118.16 - 0.163 \times$ yrs $- 0.0937 \times$ cm; RSD = 3.11
   $FEF_{25-75\%}$ (L/sec) = $+2.683 - 0.0460 \times$ yrs $+ 0.0154 \times$ cm; RSD = 0.792

4. Crapo RO, Morris AH, Clayton PD, et al. Lung volumes in healthy nonsmoking adults. *Bull Europ Physiopath Resp*. 1982;18:419–25.

   Men
   TLC (L) = $-7.333 + 0.0032 \times$ yrs $+ 0.0795 \times$ cm; RSD = 0.792
   FRC (L) = $-5.290 + 0.0090 \times$ yrs $+ 0.0472 \times$ cm; RSD = 0.718
   RV (L) = $-2.840 + 0.0207 \times$ yrs $+ 0.0216 \times$ cm; RSD = 0.374
   RV/TLC (%) = $+14.06 + 0.3090 \times$ yrs; RSD = 4.38

   Women
   TLC (L) = $-4.537 + 0.0590 \times$ cm; RSD = 0.536
   FRC (L) = $-3.182 + 0.0031 \times$ yrs $+ 0.0360 \times$ cm; RSD = 0.523

RV (L) = $-$ 2.421 + 0.0201 $\times$ yrs + 0.0197 $\times$ cm; RSD = 0.381
RV/TLC (%) = +14.35 + 0.4160 $\times$ yrs; RSD = 5.46

5. Gutierrez C, Ghezzo RH, Abboud RT, et al. Reference values of pulmonary function tests for Canadian Caucasians. *Can Respir J.* 2004;11:414–24.

Men

TLC (L) = $-$ 8.618 + 0.090 $\times$ cm; RSD = 0.817
VC (L) = $-$ 5.897– 0.023 $\times$ yrs + 0.069 $\times$ cm; RSD = 0.595
FRC (L) = $-$ 4.633 + 0.046 $\times$ cm; RSD = 0.715
RV (L) = $-$2.443 + 0.021 $\times$ yrs + 0.020 $\times$ cm; RSD = 0.470
FVC (L) = $-$ 5.473 – 0.026 $\times$ yrs + 0.067 $\times$ cm; RSD = 0.589
FEV_1 (L) = $-$ 2.832 – 0.03 $\times$ yrs + 0.047 $\times$ cm; RSD = 0.500
FEV_1/FVC (%) = + 109.396 – 0.21 $\times$ yrs – 0.113 $\times$ cm; RSD = 5.821
DLCO (mL/min/mmHg) = $-$ 4.625 – 0.246 $\times$ yrs + 0.284 $\times$ cm; RSD = 5.368
DLVO/VA' = + 10.305 – 0.031 $\times$ yrs – 0.023 $\times$ cm; RSD = 0.701
RV/TLC none

Women

TLC (L) = $-$ 5.965 – 0.007 $\times$ yrs + 0.071 $\times$ cm; RSD = 0.583
VC (L) = $-$ 3.597 – 0.021 $\times$ yrs + 0.050 $\times$ cm; RSD = 0.470
FRC (L) = $-$ 3.573 + 0.039 $\times$ cm; RSD = 0.469
RV (L) = $-$2.314 + 0.015 $\times$ yrs + 0.020 $\times$ cm; RSD = 0.378
FVC (L) = $-$ 3.335 – 0.024 $\times$ yrs + 0.049 $\times$ cm; RSD = 0.427
FEV_1 (L) = $-$ 1.901 – 0.025 $\times$ yrs + 0.037 $\times$ cm; RSD = 0.340
FEV_1/FVC (%) = + 104.509 – 0.182 $\times$ yrs – 0.089 $\times$ cm; RSD = 5.68
DLCO (mL/min/mmHg) = $-$ 7.781 – 0.153 $\times$ yrs + 0.236 $\times$ cm; RSD = 3.469
DLCO/VA' = + 5.200 – 0.014 $\times$ yrs; RSD = 0.697
RV/TLC none

6. Hankinson JL, Odenkranz JR, Fedan KB. Spirometric reference values from a sample of the general US population. *Am J Respir Crit Care Med.* 1999;179–87.

Wh men	Constant	Yrs	Yrs^2	Mean cm^2	LLN cm^2
FEV_1 (L)	0.5536	–0.01303	–0.00017	0.000141	0.000116
FEV_6 (L)	0.1102	–0.00842	–0.00022	0.000182	0.000153
FVC (L)	–0.1933	0.00064	–0.00027	0.000186	0.000157
PEF (L/s)	1.0523	0.08272	–0.0013	0.00025	0.000176
25–75%	2.7006	–0.04995		0.000103	5.29E–05
Bl men	Constant	Yrs	Yrs^2	Mean cm^2	LLN cm^2
FEV_1 (L)	0.3411	–0.02309		0.000132	0.000106
FEV_6 (L)	–0.0547	–0.02114		0.000164	0.000135
FVC (L)	–0.1517	–0.01821		0.000166	0.000137
PEF (L/s)	222.57	–0.04082		0.000273	0.000189
25–75%	2.1477	–0.04238		0.000105	4.82E–05

Lat men	Constant	Yrs	Yrs^2	Mean cm^2	LLN cm^2
FEV$_1$ (L)	0.6306	−0.02928		0.000151	0.000127
FEV$_6$ (L)	0.5757	−0.0286		0.000178	0.00015
FVC (L)	0.2376	−0.00891	−0.00018	0.000178	0.000149
PEF (L/s)	0.087	0.0658	−0.0012	0.000302	0.000218
25–75%	1.7503	−0.05018		0.000145	9.02E−05
Wh Wom	Constant	Yrs	Yrs^2	Mean cm^2	LLN cm^2
FEV$_1$	0.4333	−0.00361	−0.00019	0.000115	9.28E−05
FEV$_6$	−0.1373	0.01317	−0.00035	0.000144	0.000118
FVC	−0.356	0.0187	−0.00038	0.000148	0.000122
PEF(L/s)	0.9267	0.06929	−0.00103	0.000186	0.000121
25–75%	2.367	−0.01904	−0.0002	6.98E−05	2.3E−05
Bl Wom	Constant	Yrs	Yrs^2	Mean cm^2	LLN cm^2
FEV$_1$	0.3433	−0.01283	−9.7E−05	0.000108	8.55E−05
FEV$_6$	−0.1981	0.000047	−0.00023	0.000135	0.000108
FVC	−0.3039	0.00536	−0.00027	0.000136	0.000109
PEF(L/s)	1.3597	0.03458	−0.00085	0.000197	0.000122
25–75%	2.0828	−0.00379		8.57E−05	3.38E−05
Lat Wom	Constant	Yrs	Yrs^2	Mean cm^2	LLN cm^2
FEV$_1$	0.4529	−0.01178	−0.00011	0.000122	9.89E−05
FEV$_6$	0.2033	0.0002	−0.00023	0.000141	0.000115
FVC	0.121	0.00307	−0.00024	0.000142	0.000116
PEF (L/s)	0.2401	0.06174	−0.00102	0.000222	0.000146
25–75%	1.7456	−0.01195	−0.00029	9.61E−05	4.59E−05

Wh Men	Yrs	Mean Constant	LLN Constant
FEV$_1$/FEV$_6$,%	−0.1382	87.34	78.372
FEV$_1$/FVC,%	−0.20666	88.066	78.388
Bl Men	Yrs	Mean Constant	LLN Constant
FEV$_1$/FEV$_6$,%	−0.1305	88.841	78.979
FEV$_1$/FVC,%	−0.1828	89.239	78.822
Lat Men	Yrs	Mean Constant	LLN Constant
FEV$_1$/FEV$_6$,%	−0.1534	89.388	80.81
FEV$_1$/FVC,%	−0.2186	90.024	80.925
Wh Wom	Yrs	Mean Constant	LLN Constant
FEV$_1$/FEV$_6$,%	−0.1563	90.107	81.307
FEV$_1$/FVC,%	−0.2125	90.809	81.015

Bl Wom	Yrs	Mean Constant	LLN Constant
FEV$_1$/FEV$_6$,%	−0.1558	91.229	81.396
FEV$_1$/FVC,%	−0.2039	91.655	80.978
Lat Wom	Yrs	Mean Constant	LLN Constant
FEV$_1$/FEV$_6$,%	−0.167	91.664	83.034
FEV$_1$/FVC,%	−0.2248	92.36	83.044

7. Hankinson JL, Crapo RO, Jensen RL. Spirometric reference values for the 6–s FVC maneuver. *Chest*. 2003;124:1805–11.

Men

Constant	Yrs	Yrs^2	Mean cm^2	LLN cm^2
FEV$_6$ (L) White = 0.077	−0.00717	−0.0002353	0.0001819	0.0001531
FEV$_6$ (L) Black = −0.163	−0.1540	0.0077730	0.0001638	0.00013468
FEV$_6$ (L) Latin = 0.401	−0.019	−0.0001022	0.0001783	0.00015043
FEV$_3$ (L) White = 0.403	−0.02000	−0.0001365	0.0001758	0.00014784
FEV$_3$ (L) Black = 0.252	+0.0350	0.0001177	0.0001593	0.00013085
FEV$_3$ (L) Latin = 0.537	−0.0280	−0.0000394	0.0001751	0.00014811

FEV$_1$/FEV$_6$ (%) White = 87.36 − 0.139 × yrs; RSD = 5.51
FEV$_1$/FEV$_6$ (%) Black = 88.72 − 0.128 × yrs; RSD = 6.01
FEV$_1$/FEV$_6$ (%) Latin = 89.22 − 0.150 × yrs; RSD = 5.29

Women

Constant	Yrs	Yrs^2	Mean cm^2	LLN cm^2
FEV$_6$ (L) White = −0.187	0.01200	−0.0003453	0.0001464	0.00012151
FEV$_6$ (L) Black = −0.192	0.00080	−0.0002330	0.0001344	0.00010837
FEV$_6$ (L) Latin = 0.222	−0.00018	−0.0002257	0.0001407	0.00011451
FEV$_3$ (L) White = 0.085	0.00340	−0.0002776	0.0001407	0.00011668
FEV$_3$ (L) Black = −0.011	−0.00655	−0.0001726	0.0001307	0.00010540
FEV$_3$ (L) Latin = 0.364	−0.00611	−0.0001826	0.0001370	0.00011160

FEV$_1$/FEV$_6$ (%) White = 90.19 − 0.159 × yrs; RSD = 5.30
FEV$_1$/FEV$_6$ (%) Black = 91.19 − 0.156 × yrs; RSD = 6.09
FEV$_1$/FEV$_6$ (%) Latin = 91.71 − 0.170 × yrs; RSD = 5.33

8. Hansen JE, Sun XG, Wasserman K. Discriminating measures and normal values for expiratory obstruction. *Chest*. 2006;129:369–77.

Men

White FEV$_1$/FVC (%) = +86.03 − 0.160 × yrs; RSD = 6.00
Black FEV$_1$/FVC (%) = +89.87 − 0.2016 × yrs; RSD = 5.84

Latin FEV_1/FVC (%) = +89.09 − 0.1947 × yrs; RSD = 5.38
All men FEV_1/FVC (%) = +88.38 − 0.1952 × yrs; RSD = 6.09

Women
White FEV_1/FVC (%) = +90.84 − 0.2116 × yrs; RSD = 5.81
Black FEV_1/FVC (%) = +91.21 − 0.1936 × yrs; RSD = 6.38
Latin FEV_1/FVC (%) = +91.24 − 0.2029 × yrs; RSD = 5.65
All women FEV_1/FVC (%) = +91.11 − 0.2030 × yrs; RSD = 6.16

Men
White FEV_3/FVC (%) = +100.63 − 0.1692 × yrs; RSD = 3.42
Black FEV_3/FVC (%) = +100.99 − 0.1699 × yrs; RSD = 3.02
Latin FEV_3/FVC (%) = +101.02 − 0.1773 × yrs; RSD = 2.70
All men FEV_3/FVC (%) = +100.86 − 0.1756 × yrs; RSD = 3.22

Women
White FEV_3/FVC (%) = +102.41 − 0.1826 × yrs; RSD = 3.57
Black FEV_3/FVC (%) = +100.86 − 0.1568 × yrs; RSD = 3.46
Latin FEV_3/FVC (%) = +101.74 − 0.1740 × yrs; RSD = 3.01
All women FEV_3/FVC (%) = +101.83 − 0.1782 × yrs; RSD = 3.53

9. Hansen JE, Sun XG, Wasserman K. Ethnic– and sex–free formulae for detection of airway obstruction. *Am Rev Respir Crit Care Med.* 2006;174:493–8.

Men and women of three ethnicities.

FEV_1/FVC (%) = +98.8 − 0.25 × yrs − 1.79 × FVC (L); RSD = 5.70,
FEV_3/FVC (%) = +105.4 − 0.20 × yrs − 0.75 × FVC (L); RSD = 3.19

10. Hansen JE, Sun XG, Wasserman K. Should forced expiratory volume in six seconds replace forced vital capacity to detect airway obstruction? *Eur Respir J.* 2006; 27:1–8.

Men
Black FEV_3/FEV_6 (%) = 99.31 − 0.0815 × yrs; RSD = 2.16, r^2 = 0.239
Latin FEV_3/FEV_6 (%) = 99.81 − 0.0942 × yrs; RSD = 1.64, r^2 = 0.416
White FEV_3/FEV_6 (%) = 99.38 − 0.0842 × yrs; RSD = 1.85, r^2 = 0.396
All men FEV_3/FEV_6 (%) = 99.5 − 0.0865 × yrs; RSD = 1.86, r^2 = 0.367

Women
Black FEV_3/FEV_6 (%) = 99.94 − 0.0867 × yrs; RSD = 2.09, r^2 = 0.305
Latin FEV_3/FEV_6 (%) = 100.29 − 0.0958 × yrs; RSD = 1.82, r^2 = 0.406
White FEV_3/FEV_6 (%) = 100.69 − 0.1026 × yrs; RSD = 2.06, r^2 = 0.442
All women FEV_3/FEV_6 (%) = 100.32 − 0.0958 × yrs; RSD = 2.00, r^2 = 0.411

11. Hansen JE, Sun XG. Both genders and three ethnicities from never–smoking NHANES–3 adults using only age and FVC or FEV_6 values. Unpublished 2009.
FEV_1/FVC (%) = 99.37− 0.256 × yrs − 1.88 × FVC (L); RSD = 5.67, r^2 = 0.323
FEV_3/FVC (%) = 104.69 − 0.192 × yrs − 0.67 × FVC (L); RSD = 3.23, r^2 =0.465

$FEV_1/FEV_6 (\%) = 96.58 - 0.182 \times yrs - 1.54 \times FEV_6 (L); RSD = 5.04, r^2 = 0.225$
$FEV_3/FEV_6 (\%) = 101.40 - 0.100 \times yrs - 0.29 \times FEV_6 (L); RSD = 1.86, r^2 = 0.414$

12. Hansen JE, Sun XG. Using age and height from 760 NHANES–3 never–smoking white men and 1400 never–smoking white women. Unpublished 2010.

Men
$FVC (L) = -5.396 - 0.0261 \times yrs + 0.0657 \times cm; RSD = 0.591, r^2 = 0.581$
$FEV_1 (L) = -2.639 - 0.0286 \times yrs + 0.0447 \times cm; RSD = 0.493, r^2 = 0.623$
$FEV_3 (L) = -4.362 - 0.0327 \times yrs + 0.05958 \times cm; RSD = 0.548, r^2 = 0.659$
$FEV_6 (L) = -4.889 - 0.0301 \times yrs + 0.0631 \times cm; RSD = 0.566, r^2 = 0.631$
$FEV_1/FVC (\%) = +111.6 - 0.17 \times yrs - 0.142 \times cm; RSD = 5.75\%; r^2 = 0.205$
$FEV_1/FEV_6 (\%) = +108.2 - 0.095 \times yrs - 0.129 \times cm; RSD = 5.05\%, r^2 = 0.108$
$FEV_3/FEV_6 (\%) = +102.5 - 0.084 \times yrs - 0.018 \times cm; RSD = 1.49, r^2 = 0.376$
$FEV_3/FVC (\%) = +107.0 - 0.172 \times yrs - 0.035 \times cm; RSD = 3.06; r^2 = 0.438$

Women
$FVC (L) = -3.387 - 0.0201 \times yrs + 0.04798 \times cm; RSD = 0.427; r^2 = 0.628$
$FEV_1 (L) = -1.568 - 0.0239 \times yrs + 0.03376 \times cm; RSD = 0.346; r^2 = 0.711$
$FEV_3 (L) = -2.614 - 0.02537 \times yrs + 0.043454 \times cm; RSD = 0.393; r^2 = 0.708$
$FEV_6 (L) = -3.044 - 0.023 \times yrs + 0.0462 \times cm; RSD = 0.413; r^2 = 0.670$
$FEV_1/FEV_6 (\%) = +109.6 - 0.197 \times yrs - 0.041 \times cm; RSD = 3.62\%; r^2 = 0.468$
$FEV_1/FVC (\%) = +111.8 - 0.238 \times yr - 0.124 \times cm; RSD = 5.77\%; r^2 = 0.322$
$FEV_3/FEV_6 (\%) = +104.7 - 0.106 \times yr - 0.024 \times cm; RSD = 1.96\%; r^2 = 0.462$
$FEV_3/FVC (\%) = +108.0 - 0.162 \times yr - 0.111 \times cm; RSD = 4.96\%, r^2 = 0.227$

13. Knudson RJ, Lebowitz MD, Holberg CJ. Changes in the normal maximal expiratory flow–volume curve with growth and aging. *Am Rev Respir Dis.* 1983;127:725–34.

Men >25 yrs
$FVC (L) = -8.782 + 0.0844 \times cm - 0.0298 \times yrs; RSD = 0.638$
$FEV_1 (L) = -6.515 + 0.0665 \times cm - 0.0292 \times yrs; RSD = 0.524$
$FEV_1/FVC (\%) = +86.69 - 0.1050 \times yrs; RSD = 6.27$
$FEV_1/FVC (\%) = +96.3 - 0.1677 \times yrs - 1.4232 \times FVC (L); RSD = 6.183$
$FEF_{25-75\%} (L/sec) = -4.518 - 0.0363 \times yrs + 0.0579 \times cm; RSD = 1.082$

Women > 20 yrs
$FVC (L) = -2.9 + 0.0427 \times cm - 0.0174 \times yrs; RSD = 0.483$
$FEV_1 (L) = -1.405 + 0.0309 \times cm - 0.0201 \times yrs; RSD = 0.390$
$FEV_1/FVC (\%) = +121.68 - 0.1896 \times yrs - 0.1852 \times cm; RSD = 7.570$
$FEV_1/FVC (\%) = +113.69 - 0.2904 \times yrs - 5.4024 \times FVC (L); RSD = 7.048$
$FEF_{25-75\%} (L/sec) = -0.4057 - 0.0309 \times yrs + 0.030 \times cm; RSD = 0.854$

14. Miller A, Thornton JC, Warshaw R, et al. Single breath diffusing capacity in a representative sample of the population of Michigan, a large industrial state. Predicted values, lower limits of normal, and frequencies of abnormality by smoking history. *Am Rev Respir Dis.* 1983;127:270–7.

Men

DLCO (mL/min/mmHg) = 13.05 + 0.164 × cm − 0.23 × yrs

Women

DLCO (mL/min/mmHg) = 0.65 + 0.16 × cm − 0.11 × yrs

15. Miller MR, Grove DM, Pincock AC. Time domain spirogram indices. Their variability and reference values in nonsmokers. *Am Rev Respir Dis*. 1985;132:1041–8.

Men

FVC (L) = − 5.16 − 0.018 × yrs + 0.0612 × cm; RSD = 0.47
FEV_1 (L) = − 2.28 − 0.030 × yrs + 0.0419 × cm; RSD = 0.42
FEV_3 (L) = − 4.01 − 0.031 × yrs + 0.0563 × cm; RSD= 0.44
FEV_1/FVC (%) = +128.2 − 0.201 × yrs; RSD = 5.99
FEV_3/FVC (%) = +102.8 − 0.191 × yrs; RSD= 3.05

Women

FVC (L) = − 3.01 − 0.018 × yrs + 0.0444 × cm; RSD = 0.34
FEV_1 (L) = − 1.36 − 0.026 × yrs + 0.0325 × cm; RSD = 0.30
FEV_3 (L) = − 2.55 − 0.032 × yrs + 0.0446 × cm; RSD = 0.33
FEV_1/FVC (%) = +95.8 − 0.32 × yrs; RSD = 5.45
FEV_3/FVC (%) = +107.8 − 0.271 × yrs; RSD = 3.13

16. Paoletti P, Pistelli G, Fazzi P, et al. Reference values for vital capacity and flow volume curves from a general population study. *Bull Eur Physiopathol Respir*. 1986;22:451–9.

Men

FEV_1 (L) = − 3.576 − 0.0275 × yrs + 0.0494 × cm; RSD = 0.48
FVC (L) = − 6.382 − 0.027 × yrs + 0.0724 × cm; RSD = 0.58

Women

FEV_1 (L) = − 0.282 − 0.020 × yrs + 0.0243 × cm; RSD = 0.29
FVC (L) = − 2.329 − 0.015 × yrs + 0.0412 × cm; RSD = 0.38

17. Quanjer PH, Tammeling GJ, Cotes JE, et al. Lung volumes and ventilatory flows. *Eur Respir J*. 1993;6(Suppl.16):5–40.

Men

(if below age 25, use 25 rather than actual age)
IVC (L) = − 4.65 − 0.028 × yrs + 0.061 × cm; RSD = 0.56
FVC (L) = − 4.34 − 0.026 × yrs + 0.0576 × cm; RSD = 0.61
FEV_1 (L) = − 2.49 − 0.029 × yrs + 0.043 × cm; RSD = 0.51
FEV_1/VC (%) = + 87.21 − 0.18 × yrs; RSD = 7.17
TLC (L) = − 7.08 + 0.0799 × cm; RSD = 0.70
RV (L) = − 1.23+0.022 × yrs + 0.0131 × cm; RSD = 0.41
FRC (L) = − 1.09+ 0.01 × yrs + 0.0234 × cm; RSD = 0.60
FRC/TLC (%) = +43.8 + 0.21 × yrs; RSD = 6.74%

RV/TLC (%) = +14.0 + 0.39 × yrs; RSD = 5.46%

ERV (L) = Pred FRC – Pred RV

Women

(if below age 25, use 25 rather than actual age)

IVC (L) = – 3.28 – 0.026 × yrs + 0.0468 × cm; RSD = 0.42

FVC (L) = – 2.89 – 0.026 × yrs + 0.0443 × cm; RSD = 0.43

FEV_1 (L) = – 2.60 – 0.025 × yrs + 0.0395 × cm; RSD = 0.38

FEV_1/VC (%) = + 89.10 – 0.19 × yrs; RSD = 6.51

TLC (L) = – 5.79 + 0.066 × cm; RSD = 0.60

RV (L) = – 2.00 + 0.016 × yrs + 0.0181 × cm; RSD = 0.35

FRC (L) = – 1.00 + 0.001 × yrs + 0.0224 × cm; RSD = 0.50

FRC/TLC (%) = +45.1 + 0.16 × yrs; RSD = 5.93%

RV/TLC (%) = +19.0 + 0.34 × yrs; RSD = 5.83%

ERV (L) = Pred FRC – Pred RV

18. Roca J, Sanchis J, Agusti–Videl A, et al. Spirometric reference values for a Mediterranean population. *Bull Eur Physiopathol Respir.* 1986;22:451–9.

Men

FVC (L) = – 6.055 – 0.0147 × yrs + 0.067811 × cm; RSD= 0.53

FEV_1 (L) = – 3.955 – 0.0216 × yrs + 0.0514 × cm; RSD = 0.45

FEV_1/FVC (%) = 84–6%

Women

FVC (L) = – 2.825 – 0.0211 × yrs + 0.0454 × cm; RSD= 0.40

FEV_1 (L) = – 1.286 – 0.0253 × yrs + 0.0326 × cm; RSD = 0.32

FEV_1/FVC (%) = 82–7%

Appendix C
Abbreviations, Symbols and Definitions

Note: Abbreviations used only in specific tables or figures, are not listed below.

ABBREVIATIONS AND SYMBOLS

ATP	= adenosine tri-phosphate
ATS	= American Thoracic Society
BD	= bronchodilator, aerosolized, in laboratory
BMI	= body mass index, kg/m^2
BTPS	= body temperature pressure saturated (at ambient pressure and usually at 37°C, saturated with pH_2O of 47 mmHg).
BR	= breathing reserve
CaO_2	= content of oxygen in arterial blood, usually mL/dL
CvO_2	= content of oxygen in mixed-venous blood, usually mL/dL
$C(a\text{-}v)O_2$	= difference between content of oxygen in arterial and mixed-venous blood
CB	= chronic bronchitis
CH_4	= methane
CHO	= carbohydrate
CO	= carbon monoxide
CO_2	= carbon dioxide
COHgb	= carboxyhemoglobin
COPD	= chronic obstructive pulmonary disease
COV	= coefficient of variation
CP	= creatine phosphate
CPET	= cardiopulmonary exercise test with gas exchange and cardiovascular measurements
DLCO	= diffusing capacity of the lung for carbon monoxide
ERS	= European Respiratory Society
ERV	= expiratory reserve volume
$FACO_2$, $FECO_2$, $FICO_2$	= fractional concentration of CO_2 (or other gas) in alveolar, mixed-expired, or inspired volumes
FEV_1	= forced expiratory volume in one second
FEV_3	= forced expiratory volume in three seconds
FEV_6	= forced expiratory volume in six seconds
$FEF_{25\text{-}75\%}$	= mean forced expiratory flow from 25–75% of FVC
FEV_x or FEV_y	= forced expiratory volumes in x and y seconds
$\%FEV_x/FEV_y$	= ratio of FEVx/FEVy, in percentage
$\%FEV_x/FVC$	= ratio of FEVx/FVC, in percentage
FRC	= functional residual capacity
FVC	= forced vital capacity

GOLD	=	Global Initiative for Chronic Obstructive Lung Disease
$[H^+]$	=	hydrogen ion
Hgb	=	hemoglobin
$[HCO_3^-]$	=	bicarbonate ion
He	=	helium
HR	=	heart rate
HRR	=	heart rate reserve
IC	=	inspiratory capacity
IRV	=	inspiratory reserve volume
IVC	=	inspiratory vital capacity
LLN	=	lower limit of normal at the 95% confidence limit
MAc	=	metabolic or non-respiratory acidosis
MAlk	=	metabolic or non-respiratory alkalosis
MEP	=	maximal expiratory pressure
MetHb	=	methemoglobin
MIP	=	maximal inspiratory pressure
mmHg	=	millimeters of mercury
MVV	=	maximal voluntary ventilation
N_2	=	nitrogen
Ne	=	neon
NHANES-3	=	Third National Health and Nutrition Evaluation Survey (in USA)
$\%\Delta N_2/L$	=	percent change in N_2/L during alveolar plateau of VC in single breath O_2 test
O_2-pulse	=	O_2 uptake per each heart beat, usually mL/beat
P-50	=	partial pressure of O_2 in mmHg at 50% saturation of hemoglobin
$PaCO_2$	=	arterial pressure of CO_2 in mmHg
$PACO_2$	=	alveolar pressure of CO_2 in mmHg
$P(a-ET)CO_2$	=	difference in partial pressure of arterial and end-tidal CO_2
PaO_2	=	arterial pressure of O_2 in mmHg
PAO_2	=	alveolar pressure of O_2 in mmHg
$P(A-a)O_2$	=	difference in alveolar - arterial pressure of O_2 in mmHg
Pb	=	barometric pressure
P_{BOX}	=	pressure in body plethysmograph "box" during panting maneuvers
pCO_2	=	partial pressure of CO_2
$PETCO_2$	=	end-tidal pressure of CO_2
$PETO_2$	=	end-tidal pressure of O_2
pH	=	negative logarithm to the base 10 of hydrogen ion concentration or pressure
pK or pKa	=	negative logarithm to the base 10 of the acid dissociation constant
Pm	=	pressure at the mouth during panting maneuvers in body plethysmograph
pO_2	=	partial pressure of O_2
r	=	correlation coefficient
RAc	=	respiratory acidosis
RAlk	=	respiratory alkalosis
rpm	=	revolutions per minute (usually of cycle pedals)

R or RER	=	respiratory exchange ratio, i.e., VCO_2/VO_2
RQ	=	respiratory quotient
RSD	=	residual standard deviation
RV	=	residual volume
SaO_2	=	saturation of arterial hemoglobin with O_2
SBO_2	=	single breath O_2 test (sometimes incorrectly called single breath N_2 test)
SD	=	standard deviation
SEE	=	standard error of the estimate
SHIP	=	study of health in Pomerania (Germany)
SpO_2	=	saturation of arterial O_2 measured by external oximeter
STPD	=	standard temperature pressure dry (0 degrees Centigrade and 760 mmHg)
SVC	=	slow or unforced vital capacity
Syx	=	standard error
TLC	=	total lung capacity
TLCO	=	transfer factor of the lung for carbon monoxide (same as DLCO)
ULN	=	upper limit of normal at the 95% confidence limit
VA'	=	effective alveolar volume
VCO_2	=	CO_2 output, usually STPD
VD	=	dead space volume
VE	=	ventilation, usually BTPS
VE/VCO_2	=	liters of ventilation (BTPS) required to eliminate 1 liter of CO_2 (STPD)
VE/VO_2	=	liters of ventilation (BTPS) required to uptake 1 liter of O_2 (STPD)
VO_2	=	O_2 uptake, usually STPD
VO_2 peak	=	peak O_2 uptake
$\Delta VO_2/\Delta WR$	=	change in O_2 uptake per change in watts of external work, usually mL/min
V/Q	=	ratio of ventilation to perfusion
VT	=	tidal volume
VTG	=	thoracic gas volume

DEFINITIONS OF TERMS

Acidemia	=	the pH of the blood is decreased (H^+ increased)
Acidosis	=	a process which increases [H^+]
Airspace	=	exchanges O_2 and CO_2 between the pulmonary capillaries and gas in the lung. Anatomically, from the respiratory bronchioles distally.
Airway	=	conducts air in and out of the lungs but does not exchange O_2 and CO_2. Anatomically, from the mouth and nose to the terminal bronchioles
Alkalemia	=	the pH of the blood is increased ([H^+] decreased)
Alkalosis	=	a process which decreases [H^+]
Dyspnea	=	a sensation of unusual shortness of breath
Eucapnia	=	ventilation and perfusion combine to control arterial CO_2 content within a normal range

Hypercapnia	=	arterial CO_2 content is increased
Hyperinflation	=	volume of lung is increased
Hyperoxia	=	increased O_2
Hyperventilation	=	increased ventilation of airspaces with a resultant decrease in arterial CO_2 content
Hypocapnia	=	arterial CO_2 content is reduced
Hypoventilation	=	reduced ventilation of perfused airspaces with a resultant increase in arterial CO_2 content and often with increased arterial O_2 contents.
Hypoxemia	=	reduced blood O_2 content
Hypoxia	=	decreased pO_2
Maldistribution of ventilation	=	alveolar ventilation is not well-distributed throughout the total alveolar lung volume
Non-respiratory or metabolic acidosis	=	a process causing an increase in CO_2 content and $[H^+]$
Non-respiratory or metabolic alkalosis	=	a process causing a decrease in CO_2 content and $[H^+]$
Obstructive lung disease	=	airflow is hindered on exhalation
Respiratory acidosis	=	a process causing a greater increase in arterial pCO_2 and $[H^+]$ than bicarbonate, secondary to reduced alveolar ventilation
Respiratory alkalosis	=	a process causing a greater decrease in arterial pCO_2 and $[H^+]$ than bicarbonate, secondary to increased alveolar ventilation
Restrictive lung disease	=	volume of the lung is reduced
Vascular lung disease	=	CO_2 and O_2 exchange are reduced, primarily due to low perfusion of the ventilated airspaces.

Index

Page numbers with *f* and *t* indicate figure and table respectively.